Beyond the Yeast Connection

A How-to Guide to Curing Candida and Other Yeast-Related Conditions

Warren M. Levin, M.D.
and Fran Gare, N.D.

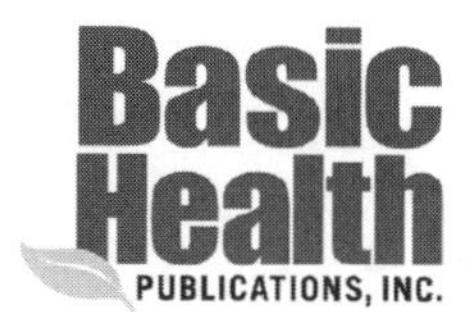

The information contained in this book is based upon the research and personal and professional experiences of the author. It is not intended as a substitute for consulting with your physician or other healthcare provider. Any attempt to diagnose and treat an illness should be done under the direction of a healthcare professional.

The publisher does not advocate the use of any particular healthcare protocol but believes the information in this book should be available to the public. The publisher and author are not responsible for any adverse effects or consequences resulting from the use of the suggestions, preparations, or procedures discussed in this book. Should the reader have any questions concerning the appropriateness of any procedures or preparation mentioned, the author and the publisher strongly suggest consulting a professional healthcare advisor.

Basic Health Publications, Inc.
28812 Top of the World Drive
Laguna Beach, CA 92651
949-715-7327 • www.basichealthpub.com

Library of Congress Cataloging-in-Publication Data is available through the Library of Congress.

Editor: Cheryl Hirsch
Typesetting/Book design: Gary A. Rosenberg
Cover design: Mike Stromberg

Printed in the United States of America

10 9 8 7 6 5 4 3 2 1

Contents

Foreword

If your doctors tell you that they can't help you, they're right. *They can't.*

But it doesn't mean you can't be helped! In fact, in my thirty-five years as a physician, I've learned that most people can be helped by holistic/integrative medicine, even when the standard medical system has failed them. This is the rule—not the exception! And this is especially so in people who have Candida-related complex (CRC), which can cause or contribute to a wide array of illnesses and symptoms, especially chronic fatigue syndrome (CFS), fibromyalgia, sinusitis, and irritable bowel syndrome—with these being just the tip of the iceberg. If these problems are present, I presume the fungus Candida (*Candida albicans*) is present and treat to eliminate it. Chronic pain in general is often also flared by Candida.

Yet, most doctors have a near-religious belief that Candida overgrowth does not even exist, unless it is so severe that it is about to kill the patient. Why? This may be because there is no reliable lab test to distinguish an overgrowth of *C. albicans* from the normal amount always present in the body. So in medicine, if there is no test, it doesn't exist! This perspective reminds me of children who cover their eyes and think that since they can't see you, you must now be invisible. This is okay for children, but it gets pretty sad when done by adults—and leaves people unnecessarily ill and often crippled. The good news? You don't have to wait for your doctors to "grow up" and open their eyes for you to get well. In fact, you can get well *now*!

Fortunately, as Dr. Levin notes in his preface, many heroes in the field have spent a lifetime laying the groundwork for our understanding of CRC. Among them is the late Dr. Billy Crook (1917–2002), one of my personal heroes and the author of *The Yeast Connection,* the landmark bestseller that introduced and familiarized the public with the Candida issue. Having done the hard work of laying the foundation, we get to expand on this work in ways that dramatically help people to get their lives back. This is what Dr. Levin excellently does here.

Fortunately, a simple questionnaire (as Dr. Levin has in this book) can help you determine if you need treatment for CRC. From there, knowledge is power, and Dr. Levin will expertly tell you how to get the Candida overgrowth eliminated. With treatment, you won't need a lab test to tell you the Candida infection is gone. Your body will tell you because you will feel so much better!

So when your doctors say they can't help you, they're right. Dr. Levin and the information in this book can! Ready to reclaim your life? Read this book! And get ready to feel great again.

Love and blessings,
Jacob Teitelbaum, M.D.

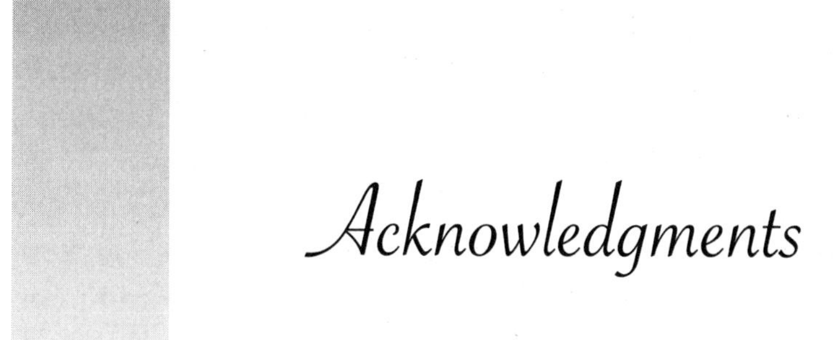

Acknowledgments

Warren Levin

After more than thirty-five years of togetherness, I must dedicate this book to Susan, my wife and partner in every part of my life since we first met. She has been urging me to write a book about my medical specialties for all those years, and I never would have done it without her.

I also want to acknowledge my mentor-colleagues, who together changed my life, my health, and very importantly my approach to the practice of medicine.

First and foremost was the great Carlton Fredericks, Ed.D., whose writings for the public led me to discover the world of nutrition. Rubbing elbows with Doctors Sid Baker, Alan Dattner, John Diamond, Alan Lieberman, Marshall Mandell, Katrina Patel, Theron Randolph, Doris Rapp, Bill Rea, Al Robbins, David Sheinkin, Butch Schrader, Francis Waickman, and many others, who banded together in the 1960s to form a field of medicine called clinical ecology, which studies how our environment affects health, has been a rare privilege. This group, which eventually founded the American Academy of Environmental Medicine (AAEM), has remained the central pillar in the foundation of my medical practice.

Other true pioneers with whom I cross-pollinated include Doctors Hyla Cass, Carol Englander, Ray Evers, Irv Goldman, Jeanne Hubboch,

John Klenner, Alan Nittler, Linus Pauling, Ivan Popov, Hy Roberts, Milton Roberts, Jacob Teitlebaum, Fred Vagnini, and Juan Wilson. I am also indebted to many members of the American College for Advancement of Medicine (ACAM), including Doctors Bob Atkins, Jeff Bland, Tammy and Grant Born, Mark Breiner, Chris Calapai, Richard Casdorph, Emanuel Cheraskin, Jonathan Collins, Elmer Cranton, Ray Evers, Jim Frackelton, Alan Gaby, Michael Gerber, Garry Gordon, Ross Gordon, Len Haimes, Bruce Halstead, Gordy Josephs, Richard Kunin, Bill Mauer, Neil Orenstein, Bob Rogers, Sherry Rogers, Glen Rothfeld, Bob Rowen, Fuller Royal, Joya Schoen, Shirley Scott, Frank Shallenberger, David Steenblock, John Toth, John Trowbridge, Robert Vance, Julian Whitaker, John Wilson, and Jonathan Wright. Doctors John Diamond, Michael Schachter, and Murray "Buz" Susser, and their respective wives Susan, Lisa, and Phyllis get special mention as best friends throughout our odyssey.

Under the tutelage of these doctors and organizations, I found great satisfaction in seeing patients with more and more complex problems, who had become more and more frustrated by mainstream medicine, which has studiously ignored the dramatic advances by those two small organizations of top-notch physicians.

In addition, with regard to Candida, special kudos go to C. Orian Truss, M.D., who published a little book in 1983 called *The Missing Diagnosis* about the role that yeasts play in many common health disorders. In it he told anyone who would listen that the problem of vaginal yeast was really started in the colon. It changed my life, my practice, and the quality of the lives of thousands of patients since that gentle tour de force. His book led to the publishing of *The Yeast Syndrome* (1986) by John Trowbridge, M.D., which mentioned me as one of the physicians who was treating the problem and gave a big boost to my practice and my confidence. Then, later that same year, came *The Yeast Connection* by Billy Crook, M.D., followed by a series of Yeast Connection books before his passing away: *The Yeast Connection Cookbook* (1989), *The Yeast Connection Handbook* (1996), *Tired—So Tired! and the Yeast Connection* (2001), and *The Yeast Connection and Women's Health* (2007), all of which helped many people, especially women, learn about this problem and its solutions.

I must also recognize several others who have played an important role in my success. These include Herman Bueno, M.D., and his first disciple Louis Parrish, M.D., from whom I learned the anoscopy method for diagnosing intestinal parasites; Rolando Cubela and Luis Cruz, who were steady fixtures on my staff; and Edith Lowinger, Esther Koven, and Barbara Newington, who were, and still are, guardian angels.

Last but not least, I want to acknowledge the members of my family, who put up with me for all these years and supported me with their love and advice: my first wife, Marsha, and our daughters Beth and Julie, and my current and last wife, Susan, and our daughter Erika. They all stayed the course and have all made me proud to be first and foremost a living "Prime Example" of what integrative medicine can do for those who choose to believe in it, follow its precepts, and fight for it.

Fran Gare

My journey into integrative medicine began as a child. My mother was a follower of nutritionist Adele Davis, and we lived according to her books. In college, my freshman orientation class was taught by Carlton Fredericks, Ed.D. His proclamations about health were frightening, yet I knew even as I sat there with my head spinning, that what he taught me would be an important part of my life's work.

When my father became ill with cancer, and traditional medicine gave up on him, I had the honor to stay with him in an alternative cancer facility, the Cancer Clinic of the late Max Gerson, M.D., in Nyack, New York. While there, I witnessed the incredible healing of tumors defecated from cancer-ridden bodies. I knew that my life's work had been sealed.

The journey has been long and exciting, learning from many important mentors in the field: Robert Atkins, M.D., who I worked with and co-authored four books with; Marshall Mandell, M.D., who I married, worked with, and co-authored two books with; Jose Rodriguez, D.C., Martin Dayton, M.D., and of course my co-author Warren Levin, M.D. Because of these men, I have had access to the pioneers in my field, calling them colleagues and friends. I thank you for your trust in me and for the respect you have shown me.

A dedication would not be complete, without acknowledging my patients, who to this day are my best teachers.

All throughout I have had the support of my family, including Ivan, Marc, and David Gare, and now their wives (Amy and Sarah), and my precious gift, Lindsay Gare, who lights up my days.

I dedicate this book to all healthcare practitioners who have come before and to those who will come after. To all who view medicine as a way for preventing illness and providing education, information, guidance, and inspiration to patients so they are able to manage their own healthcare and bring their own bodies back to healthy balance, in order to live vibrant, productive lives until the day *they decide* to leave this earth.

Preface

"Resentment is like taking poison
and waiting for the other person to die."

—MALACHY MCCOURT, IRISH-AMERICAN ACTOR AND WRITER

We are truly in charge of our own health. It is your job to tap into your body's intelligence and help it stay in balance. This book is designed to help you do that. Once you are sick, it is often too late. You are left with, "Why me?" In your mind, it could become the doctor's fault.

Doctors have many patients, and each doctor is unique in what he or she "knows" to be true—and that includes me. I have never met a doctor who didn't know something that I didn't know! I urge you to stay tenacious about your health: search for the underlying cause of your discomfort, and when you find it, locate a doctor who understands and knows how to treat the cause.

My first mentor in integrative medicine (a blending of conventional and alternative approaches) was "Dr." Carlton Fredericks—a wise and witty non-physician, whose doctorate degree was in education. He was the East Coast version of another influential non-physician on the West Coast: Adele Davis. They understood the basic fact that nutrition is applied biochemistry, and they knew a great many factoids that are still not being taught in medical schools. Carlton wrote the first book about hypoglycemia called *Low Blood Sugar and*

You (1976). In it he explained how millions of people were unknowingly suffering from this hidden disease and how a simple diet could eliminate it. That book changed the direction of my practice from mainstream medicine to what was then known as "wholistic" or "holistic" medicine (or "quackery" by the self-proclaimed "experts," who know little to nothing about the subject). Carlton mocked them, saying that the word "expert" was from ancient English with *ex* meaning "has-been" and *spurt* being "just a drip under pressure." That ignorance pitifully continues to this day.

Experts are always issuing guidelines, which are soon contradicted by another set of experts. In the medical profession, these guidelines present the "standard of care," a diagnostic and treatment process that clinicians are encouraged to follow for a certain type of patient, illness, or clinical circumstance. In most cases doctors and patients become confused by the changing guidelines, and as a result patients suffer constantly by the changing standard of care. With every new double-blind study published, a patient's care may be changed, and since most of the studies are deeply flawed, there is no agreed upon standard of care in almost anything. In my opinion, the days of "He's a doctor, who am I to question him?" should be long gone.

In reality, doctors practice according to their own individual paradigm, which they acquire over a lifetime from parents, childhood caretakers, professors, teachers, patients, and friends, and from reading, studying, and continuing to educate themselves. The most important changes in this paradigm come from each doctor's "experience" with it. Patient outcomes are our best teachers. No one is perfect. Carlton used to say, "Experience is what you get, when you were expecting something else." For that reason, the standard of care is a constantly evolving paradigm, because science is still learning the laws that govern the universe. We do not make those laws—they are what they are. You do not have to believe in the law of gravity; it has not changed since Newton was hit on the head with an apple. If it had changed, all we know about it would have had to change. Many details about it have been uncovered, argued about, understood, and applied in beneficial ways, but the law itself has not changed. So, if you jump out of window a thousand times, whether you believe in gravity or not, you will fall down—not sideways, or up—always down. There are not many things in medicine that are "set in stone" as it is with gravity. Medical care is constantly evolving, and astute physicians stay current, and individualize their treatment for the patient's best good.

Each physician's paradigm represents his or her personal philosophy, but very few have attempted to write it down. This may be because it is always changing; changing with the latest medical discoveries and each doctor's clinical experience prescribing the treatment. I was given the unusual opportunity of having to write mine down by two colleagues, who were collaborating on a textbook about nutrition and its critical function in medicine, and who had asked me to write the foreword. This important book by Russell Jaffe, M.D., and Paul Yanick, Ph.D., was subsequently published in 1988 as *Clinical Chemistry and Nutrition Guidebook.* I did not realize it then, but this foreword turned out to be an expression of my personal paradigm, the philosophy underlying my approach to medicine.

If this paradigm were like the paradigm followed by the majority of doctors in American medicine today, it would have had to be changed as time went on. Looking back I am proud to say that in 2013, my philosophy remains unchanged. I have no illusions about this philosophy attaining such stature as Newton's law of gravity, or Einstein's theory of relativity for that matter, but I believe it is one important working model that can and should be taught in medical schools. We have been suckered into the paradigm of "a pill for every ill." But no doctor can "fix" any other person. Not even surgeons, who do more and more complex and difficult procedures and save lives that were not savable in the recent past. Nonetheless, it is my hope that every surgeon having completed his or her task successfully would put down his tools, bow his head, and pray to the Creator with some such words as "Please, G-d, I have now done everything humanly possible for this patient, please complete the job by healing the wound that I have made."

Today we have many names for alternative medical practices. "Integrative," "functional," "complementary," "orthomolecular" medicine (all the same with different names) look for the underlying causes that contribute to the "miracle of healing" that can be addressed and corrected, so that the process may proceed unfettered. As an integrative physician, I look for vitamin, mineral, and other nutritional deficiencies, as well as chemical and environmental toxicities that may be interfering with the body's biochemistry and attempt to correct them with supplements and foods. I check for acute or chronic infections, commonly unrecognized allergies, and hormonal (endocrine) imbalances and malfunctioning neurotransmitters (brain chemicals) that can be remediated. My goal is to *modulate* rather than stimulate or suppress the immune system.

I believe the immune system operates on the Goldilocks principle. You remember the classic story of Goldilocks and the three bears? Her motto was that everything should be *just right*—not too hot, not too cold; not too slow, not too fast; not too hard, not too soft—and so too the immune system should be in balance. When it is out of balance, symptoms appear. If the immune system is out of balance, it is because it is either overactive or underactive.

The immune system functions as our interface with both the internal and external microscopic worlds. When the immune system is overactive (reacts "too much") or is underactive (reacts "too little"), its ability to defend us becomes compromised. In situations where the immune system is *overactive* and works more efficiently than it should, it can cause the body to react to external particles such as pollens or dust or animals, and result in typical allergies with inflammatory changes. Autoimmune diseases (in which the body begins attacking itself) are examples of conditions that can result from an *overactive* immune response to the body's own cells. In contrast, when the immune system is *underactive* and does not respond as promptly as it should, the body's ability to fend off disease-causing pathogens is weakened, leaving it susceptible to infections. In other instances, an *underactive* response to the body's own tissues may permit cancers.

There are many parts of the immune system, so there can be complicated interactions. For example, many individuals have experienced an upper respiratory allergy (an over-reaction), in which the inflammatory changes lead to swelling and obstruction of the sinus openings, preventing drainage. The ensuing stagnation of fluids in the sinuses can result in an infection (an under-reaction). Many times such problems arise from excessive drug therapy that interferes with the body's balancing act. The use of cortisone-type drugs to suppress simple allergic nasal symptoms can also suppress the part of the immune system that fights the infections, thus allowing the sinusitis to take hold. Prolonged use of steroids can even result in cancer or chronic infections like tuberculosis or exacerbations of dormant Lyme disease.

When all the components of the immune system have been brought back into balance, and "everything is just right," miracles can happen. A healthy immune system is number one in any healing process. I have found Candida-related complex (CRC), a term used to describe a yeast infection known as Candida, to be key to an imbalanced immune system, severely complicating all healing, and dramatically contributing to many of the complaints doctors hear in their offices. Without addressing CRC, physicians have few remedies to correct the reported maladies.

The majority of practitioners in mainstream medicine today still do not recognize the importance of an overgrowth of *Candida albicans* and multiple other species of yeast (fungi) that may result in otherwise unexplained clinical symptoms. When patients present with mood swings, chronic muscle aches and joint pain, poor memory, depression, sinus congestion, allergies, chemical sensitivities, digestive disturbances, fatigue, anxiety, or skin rashes, and the doctor can see no apparent reason for the complaints, they may not have done their Candida homework. They may not have ordered tests that could help with an underlying diagnosis of CRC.

I have been on the forefront of integrative medicine for forty plus years. I began testing for and treating CRC early in my practice. I share some of my illustrative Candida "cures" in this book. Then I go "beyond" Candida to reveal my insights concerning CRC and how it can be contributing to the symptoms of a wide range of such debilitating diseases as acne, autism, chronic fatigue, depression, infertility, Lyme disease, and poorly understood autoimmune diseases like thyroiditis (also called Hashimoto's thyroiditis).

If I am correct, and I believe I am, which is why I have written this book, most cases of CRC can be prevented, while not all can be completely cured. Hold on to your hats—we've got quite a ride to go!

PART ONE

Getting an Accurate Diagnosis

1 Making Sense of Candida-Related Complex

"The pursuit of excellence is gratifying and healthy. The pursuit of perfection is frustrating, neurotic, and a terrible waste of time."

—EDWIN BLISS, AUTHOR AND BUSINESS CONSULTANT

For readers who may not know me, I am Warren M. Levin, M.D. I practice integrative medicine in Virginia and have been in practice for over forty-five years. Integrative medicine is a practice of medicine that combines mainstream medical therapies with evidence-based non-conventional complementary therapies. In that time I have seen at least 50,000 patients, and in many cases, generations of patients from the same families. In my practice, we strive for excellence.

In my many years of practice, I have found that there are a few underlying health problems, often not diagnosed, that slowly destroy your health. You end up with symptoms that physicians have no explanation for, and often you are told, "It's in your head." However, what may be in your head, begins in your body.

Have you ever had a friend or family member with cancer or some other serious health condition, confide that they do not know what they could have done wrong that made them so ill? As a doctor I have heard, "I eat so healthfully. I exercise regularly, meditate, and take nutrients. Why me?"

While the answer to that question could be many things, my first thought is: a compromised or weakened immune system. The health condition could be genetic, but more likely it is due to an underlying, undiagnosed infection that is weakening the immune system and allowing disease to flourish. In many cases, that infection is Candida.

WHAT IS CANDIDA-RELATED COMPLEX?

Candida-related complex, or CRC, is caused by infection with *Candida albicans* (referred to hereafter as Candida), a common yeast belonging to a group of organisms called fungi. Candida is found in nearly everyone, and in small amounts contributes to good health. Candida is also among the most prolific yeast organisms in the human body. It grows luxuriously in warm, dark, and moist places like the nose, throat, mouth, intestinal tract, and genital areas, as long as sugar (a favorite food) is available for its growth and development.

Yeast begins its life in humans by being swallowed. It makes its way into our gastrointestinal tracts—where all those ideal conditions exist—and the organism initially grows into a lush colony in the food stream supplied during the digestive process. Contained within the gastrointestinal tract, the yeast is still "outside the body." Like a marble rolling through the cardboard center of a roll of paper towels, Candida goes in one end (the mouth) and out the other (the anus) without entering the paper (the tissues, organs, and systems) of the body. At this stage, the yeast is not invasive.

Eventually, however, as the Candida grows and multiplies, it adheres to the intestinal mucosa (the lining of the intestines), where it reproduces by budding. Here in the fungal stage, it begins sending long, filamentous roots through the intestinal lining, creating a major breach in the body's protective (paper) envelope, while anchoring itself in self-defense against the body's attempts to eliminate it. The Candida is now a parasitic organism, taking its nutrients from body fluids, rather than food waste, and giving nothing of value in return. These colonies of Candida produce powerful toxins (waste products from their own metabolic processes) that also invade the bloodstream. Once Candida and its toxic byproducts become systemic, they can infect any tissue, organ, and system in the body and cause a host of associated conditions and disorders that will gradually increase in number and severity over time—hence, the term Candida-related complex.

Dandelions of the Intestines

Yeast organisms are always present in the intestines, or gut. I call them the dandelions of the intestines. They are quick to seize the opportunity to grow and they compete successfully with the healthy bacteria in the intestines. The body requires tens of billions of these protective bacteria to be present in the gut to maintain balance and keep the Candida and other potentially harmful organisms under control. Candida is a yeast that kills healthy bacteria, destroying the balance of gut flora. Without the presence of these healthy bacteria, the yeast is free to grow, and in a sense, take over the body.

The immune system is our major defense against illness. It is important to keep it healthy and strong. Research has found that 70 to 80 percent of the immune system is located in the intestinal tract. This should not be surprising considering that the walls of the intestines have to protect against every internal and external pathogenic substance that finds its way into our gut. As the Candida colonizes and attaches to the gut mucosa, it irritates and breaks down the lining. This damage is the first step to immune dysfunction as it causes inflammation in the intestinal tract, making it impossible for needed nutrients to be used by the body. The result is a host of immune-deficient, degenerative diseases (most commonly cancer, diabetes, and heart disease) that cause our bodies to age, become ill, and die. CRC is a major cause of inflammation in the intestinal tract.

The first place I always look for a Candida infection is in the intestines, especially if the patient has had many rounds of antibiotics in her or his lifetime or has complained of recurring vaginal and urinary tract infections, indigestion, gas, itching in the vaginal and anal areas, and unexplained skin rashes. (Chapter 2 explores these conditions in greater depth.)

Benefits of Healthy Bacteria

In addition to keeping troublesome yeasts like Candida in check, healthy bacteria have other important functions. Good bacteria in the intestinal tract help us digest food. They break down fibers and other larger molecules into smaller, more bioavailable nutrients that the body can use. They make vitamins such as vitamin A, B_{12}, and K from the foods we eat that are then absorbed into our bodies through the small and large intestines.

These beneficial bacteria also help us to eliminate wastes and other toxins. They make up about 50 percent of the dry weight of a healthy stool, improve peristalsis, and help normalize bowel transit time. Yeasts, which destroy beneficial bacteria, can penetrate the intestinal walls, invading the body, and not be found in the stool because they have become systemic and are now inside the body, rather than exiting the body in fecal matter.

Healthy bacteria also help protect us against infection. They are our first defense against foreign organisms entering the body. I like using the metaphor of a healthy lawn to describe these bacteria. If you cultivate your lawn for a couple of years, buy fine top soil and spread it, till the soil, fertilize it, aerate it, lime it, water it, seed it, and weed it by hand, you end up with a beautiful network of roots. There are no weeds in a healthy lawn. You can even blow dandelion seeds (like Candida) on a lawn this healthy and although they may sprout, they will not root. Think of the lawn as a carpet of healthy bacteria in the intestines. Opportunistic infections, pathogenic bacteria, and other foreign organisms cannot invade it. Good bacteria have been shown to produce antibiotic substances that prevent foreigners from growing. It is healthy gut flora that does all of this for us, and prevents yeast organisms that come through the intestinal tract from taking hold.

WHERE YEASTS COME FROM

Yeasts are everywhere, all around us, all the time. They are found in the air, in the soil, in the water, on the surface of plants, on the human skin, and on leftover food. They contaminate the foods we eat and the water we drink, and as they go through the digestive system are destroyed by stomach acids, digestive enzymes, and the presence of adequate healthy bacteria in the gut. Some types of yeast are of great importance to humans. For example, yeast is necessary to make leavened bread, beer, cheese, vinegar, wine and other fermented products. A normally benign yeast like Candida only starts to cause trouble when it is allowed to grow out of control.

Triggers of Yeast Growth

The most common triggers of Candida overgrowth are the use of antibiotics and the consumption of sugar.

Antibiotic drugs simultaneously kill both harmful and helpful bacteria, leaving the intestinal tract wide open for opportunistic organisms to move in. The result is similar to getting brown spots in your lawn, places that allow weeds to grow. In the intestines, the first weeds to grow are Candida yeast organisms. Prolonged or repeated use of antibiotics makes it increasingly difficult for the gut to regain a healthy balance. Other widely used medications like birth control pills, stomach acid–suppressing drugs, and steroids and other anti-inflammatories also change the balance of the intestinal tract, kill the healthy bacteria that keep Candida in check, and allow it to flourish. Long-term use of these drugs causes damage to the intestinal lining, which in turn causes more inflammation, further impairing the immune system, weakening it further.

The typical Western diet provides Candida with an ideal environment in which to grow and develop. Yeasts thrive on sugar and refined processed foods, such as soft drinks, desserts, candy, baked goods, and snack foods, that can be easily broken down to sugar. When eaten in excess, over a period of many years, these foods contribute to Candida overgrowth. The digestive enzyme, amylase, begins the digestive process. As the sugar reaches the stomach, it begins a fermentation process that causes yeast bacteria to proliferate in the gut, killing healthy bacteria as it grows.

THE EFFECTS OF YEAST OVERGROWTH

The tremendous increase in yeast infections over the past fifty years is attributable to this overuse of antibiotics and certain medications, and the overconsumption of sugar. These increased opportunities make it easier for Candida to proliferate and spread, and turn from a localized noninvasive yeast infection into a chronic invasive infection, capable of producing a wide variety of diseases.

CRC is not an illness or disease per se. Rather it is a syndrome that plays a central role in a multitude of chronic, degenerative diseases and disease syndromes. Why a syndrome? A syndrome is a grouping of complaints that relate to the same underlying problem—in this case, infection by Candida.

Here is a classic example, and the one most think of when they think of a yeast infection. Twenty-seven-year-old Cynthia came to me with a recurring vaginal yeast infection that did not clear up after repeated treatment with topical antibiotics, fungal douches, creams, salves, suppositories, and ointments. I realized that the yeast had to be more than just in her vagina. When I tested it, the yeast had invaded her intestinal tract as well, and since the anus and vagina are so close together, and the area between them is dark and moist (where yeast like to grow), it was very easy for the yeast to get from the rectum to the vagina, creating recurring yeast infections.

Which comes first: the chicken or the egg? Or in this case: infection in the intestines or the vagina? C. Orian Truss, M.D., the first to discover the role of yeast in disease and illness, had an enormous breakthrough in the 1970s, when he found that if he treated and eliminated the yeast from his patients' intestines, their vaginal yeast infections cleared up.

CRC can have any one of hundreds of possible symptoms. There is a litany of chronic, bothersome, incapacitating, and seemingly unsolvable, immune-suppressive health concerns that have symptoms caused by undiagnosed CRC. Constant unexplainable fatigue, brain fog, forgetfulness, bloating after meals, joint pain, rashes, constant hunger, and vaginal itching may be just some of them. Depending on the health of your immune system and your own susceptibilities, you may develop a wide variety of symptoms and health problems. This can make it difficult to know if you have CRC.

Since CRC compromises the immune system, it can be the underlying cause of many disorders. The following are the most common chronic conditions associated with CRC:

Autoimmune diseases

Ankylosing spondylitis
Rheumatoid arthritis
Scleroderma
Sjögren's syndrome
Systemic lupus erythematosus
Thyroiditis (Hashimoto's disease)

Circulatory system

Chronic tension headaches and migraines
Cold hands and feet
High or low blood pressure
Postural hypotension (a drop in blood pressure when standing, either too suddenly or too long)
Rapid or slow heart rates

Gastrointestinal system

Bloating after meals
Cholecystitis (inflammation of the gallbladder, with or without stones)
Constant hunger
Constipation
Diarrhea
Flatulence
Intestinal spasms
Irritable bowel syndrome
Itching anus

Musculoskeletal system

Hands and feet pain
Joint, muscle, ligament, and tendon pain
Spine, neck, and back pain
Any other pain, limitation of motion, and stiffness affecting the bones, joints, muscles, fascia (connective tissue), tendons, and sinews

Nervous system

Anger and irritability
Attention deficit hyperactivity disorder (ADHD)
Autism
Brain fog
Depression
Forgetfulness
Hyperactivity
Neurosis
Paranoia (delusions of persecution or grandeur)
Psychosis
Schizophrenia

Reproductive system

Abnormal bleeding
Cervicitis (inflammation of the cervix)
Endometriosis
Extreme discomfort with genital and anal itching
Infertility
Polycystic ovaries
PMS and menstrual irregularities
Vaginitis

Respiratory system

Asthma

Bronchitis
Hay fever/allergy complicated by sinusitis
Laryngitis
Otitis (ear inflammation)
Pharyngitis
Pleurisy
Pneumonia
Rhinitis (nasal inflammation with pain, discharge, and obstruction)

Skin problems

Acne
Alopecia (total or patchy hair loss)
Cradle cap
Fungal infections of the hair, nails, and skin
Infantile eczema
Psoriasis
Seborrheic dermatitis
Severe diaper rash

Urinary system

Interstitial cystitis (inflammation of the bladder)
Kidney stones
Recurring urinary tract infections

Other Symptoms and Conditions

Chronic fatigue syndrome
Excessive fatigue
Fibromyalgia
Low libido

If you are suffering from any of these chronic conditions, I challenge you to take the quiz in the next chapter. Then read on to solve your health problems.

2

Do You Have CRC?

If you have more than one of the symptoms or chronic conditions listed in Chapter 1, then I encourage you to take my Patient Quiz. Your answers, followed by my interpretation of the test results, can help you begin to understand the many ways in which CRC may be responsible for the problems your doctor may have been unable to successfully treat or explain. A short self-exam will help you further evaluate whether Candida may have visited your body and moved in.

The cases below are real people (although their real names have been changed). You will learn much more about their conditions, case histories, and outcomes following the various treatment protocols in Part Three. For the moment, think how their health problems may relate to your life or the life of a loved one. This is about you.

PATIENT QUIZ

1	Are you like Cynthia in the prior chapter, who came to me with recurring urinary tract and vaginal yeast infections that could not be cleared up with topical antibiotics?	YES	NO
2	Libby had such disturbing irritable bowel symptoms of gas, bloating, and burping that she felt self-conscious going out in public. Is this happening to you?	YES	NO

3	Brianna had severe acne and skin rashes bordering on psoriasis that she was unable to clear or control. The doctor had no explanation for them and kept treating her with antibiotics, which stopped working. Does this sound familiar to you?	YES	NO
4	Then there was the McClarity family from Florida who came to the office visit together. They were all feeling badly. All four were overweight and craved carbohydrates. They had "brain fog" (trouble thinking). Do you think this is you?	YES	NO
5	Paul was tired and depressed all of the time. He ate healthily, did his best to exercise three times a week, took vitamins, yet had trouble getting out of bed in the morning. Is something unexplained like this zapping your energy?	YES	NO
6	Nina and Philip Goldberg had a fertility problem. They had been checked at fertility clinics and were told that there wasn't any reason they should not conceive. Is there a baby in your future?	YES	NO
7	Marilyn, a vital, beautiful woman, complained of menstrual disorders and a lack of libido. She thought she was finished with passion at thirty. Do you have low libido?	YES	NO
8	Sally had been on long-term birth control pills. She went off of them so she could become pregnant, but all she could do was itch in the vaginal area. Richard, her husband, had also developed an anal itch. Do you have this scratchy problem?	YES	NO
9	Peter came to my office angry, and stayed angry the whole time he was there. We were very kind to him, but his hostile behavior did not stop. He disrupted everything, and was out of control. Do you have uncontrollable spurts of anger for no apparent reason?	YES	NO
10	I see many hyperactive children. Rosie was one of them. When questioning her parents, they reported that she was born with cradle cap and thrush (a yeast infection of the tongue and/or lips), and had infantile eczema that was treated with antibiotics. Is this somewhere in your past?	YES	NO

SCORE: If you answered YES to at least two of these questions, *read this book.* It could be your key to a healthier, happier life.

EXPLANATION OF TEST RESULTS

CRC not only manifests in an enormous variety of illnesses and symptoms, but it also affects people of each gender and all ages. While there can be many reasons for the following conditions, I often find Candida is involved.

QUESTION 1 Urinary Tract and Vaginal Infections

A urinary tract infection (UTI) can happen anywhere along the urinary tract. UTIs have different names, depending on what part of the urinary tract is infected. An infection in the bladder is called cystitis; in the kidneys, pyelonephritis; and in the urethra (the tube that empties urine from the bladder), urethritis. UTIs occur when bacteria get inside the urinary tract and multiply, causing an infection that can cause pain or burning with urination. Recurrent UTIs (generally defined as more than two infections in a six-month period) most often result from an incomplete emptying of some part of the urinary tract. Many factors can cause this: kidney stones, cysts, anatomical changes from injuries at childbirth or surgery, and congenital errors of anatomy such as hypospadias, which can cause the opening of the urethra to be pushed too far back on the underside of the penis or on the upper wall of the vagina. These and other conditions may contribute to recurrent infections, plus many of them are aggravated by sexual activity, which can move bacteria from the bowel or vaginal cavity to the urethral opening.

When not quickly treated UTIs can lead to vaginal yeast infection (vaginitis) in women, or less commonly jock itch in men. Both conditions are most often caused by an overgrowth of yeast. Vaginitis and jock itch can cause inflammation of the external genitalia, including the orifice of the urethra, which then becomes more vulnerable to external contamination with re-infection of the bladder—truly a vicious cycle.

Recurring UTIs, which are most common in women, vaginal yeast infections, and jock itch are among the most common reasons for multiple long courses of antibiotics—a major contributor to CRC.

QUESTION 2 Irritable Bowel Syndrome

CRC is a major cause of irritable bowel syndrome (IBS). Think about it. If your digestive system is compromised, how can it properly digest what you eat? The result is an unhealthy digestive tract. There are many sources of gastrointestinal (GI) upset, but gassiness is typical of CRC, especially in younger people. (Deteriorating gastrointestinal function is a common accompaniment of aging, so the gas is less specific as you age.) When you do have a Candida infection, the gas is formed by the fermentation of the sugars in the food feeding the yeast organisms. In some cases, the fermentation produces enough alcohol to cause drunken behavior, which can be evidenced by a breathalyzer test! Yeast overgrowth in the gut can cause many other non-specific GI complaints including cramps, constipation, diarrhea, irritable bowel syndrome, nausea, loss of appetite, and a burning in the stomach coming from the upper GI tract that can reflux into the esophagus (often thought of as heartburn or GERD, short for gastroesophageal reflux disease).

Most people with heartburn and GERD are treated with acid-suppressant drugs, which exacerbate the problem, since these drugs can aggravate the overgrowth of Candida. When there is not enough acid in the stomach, all kinds of harmful microorganisms which should be killed in the stomach's resting acid, get through to the small and large intestines where they find a much more comfortable place to live. A healthy stomach would have kept them out. Indeed, I have had great success in treating heartburn and GERD as a Candida problem!

QUESTION 3 Severe Acne and Skin Conditions

Another common cause of CRC is severe acne that has been treated for a year or more with antibiotics.

Antibiotics kill propionbacteria, the bacteria responsible for acne, but they also destroy many normal healthy bacteria residing in the intestines. As you already know by now, when such bacteria are wiped out, yeasts are apt to take their place. I will recommend over and over in this book what I practice as a doctor: never take antibiotics without also taking an antifungal and probiotic supplements (concentrated supplements of beneficial bacteria). Probiotics help restore the normal healthy bacteria and antifungals help inhibit the growth of Candida and others yeasts.

Psoriasis is another malady that is closely related to CRC. When CRC is successfully treated, the psoriasis generally clears, even though the active lesions do not demonstrate the presence of Candida.

QUESTION 4 Food Allergy Addiction and Overweight

The causes of poor control of appetite and weight are not well understood. Yet it's clear that sugar and refined carbohydrate cravings are rampant in the United States. This is evident by the amount of sugar consumed per person (142 pounds) a year; by the percentage of Americans who are overweight or obese (68 percent and rising); and by the number of reported cases of type 2 diabetes (26 million), a serious medical condition that affects the way the body metabolizes excess amounts of sugar (glucose).

Food allergy addiction is a common cause of overeating—especially sugar. Food allergies can cause people to crave foods to which they are allergic. Briefly, delayed food allergies (as opposed to rapid-onset severe food reactions) are much more common and more difficult to recognize. They usually develop gradually over a period of months and years and they tend to show up in people who have the proclivity for eating the same foods over and over again. Just like someone who is addicted to alcohol or drugs experiences a temporary high and suffers withdrawal symptoms when the substance is withdrawn, a person who is allergic to sugar experiences a craving for sweets, which results in overeating it for the temporary high, but eventually leads to a withdrawal reaction, causing him or her to "need" another fix.

CRC superimposes itself on this problem, because the Candida organism requires sugar for its existence and growth. Somehow it communicates this to the appetite center of the host, which significantly increases the sugar-craving signals, setting up a continuing cycle.

QUESTION 5 Excessive Fatigue and Depression

Because men rarely get UTIs and never get vaginal yeast infections, they are denied the most common external red flag to let them know they may have a Candida infection. Frequently, their first sign of CRC is feeling uncharacteristically tired and depressed. Since our bodies function as a whole, any extreme disturbance can result in a loss of energy. This is a common reaction to most any infection in the body, and Candida is an important one.

Occasionally, perhaps from optimum genital hygiene practices, a woman may have CRC with an overgrowth of Candida in the bowel yet not in the vagina. Like many men, her major complaint may start out with feeling fatigued "for no apparent reason," thus allowing the Candida to develop without being detected. I have found that in these cases, even the stool culture for yeast is negative, as the Candida has been in the system so long that it has invaded the body and is no longer present in the stool.

QUESTION 6 Infertility

Infertility is usually defined as the inability to conceive after a year or more of unprotected sexual activity. Severe Candida growth can interfere with the delicate balance of the female hormones (all three forms of estrogen, and progesterone) that control the ability to get pregnant. This hormonal imbalance shows itself most clearly with relationship to irregular ovulation, endometriosis (a buildup of excess uterine tissue), polycystic ovaries (cysts on the ovaries), and variations in the bleeding cycle from one month to another. Infertility may also be related to low levels of the thyroid hormone triiodothyronine (T3), or to an obstruction in the fallopian tubes (the passageway for the fertilized egg into the uterus) due to the Candida infection. All hormones work in tandem. When a major thyroid hormone is compromised, it affects sperm production by interfering with testosterone.

Note: If infertility is your problem, you may be able to save yourself the significant expense of fertility tests and artificial insemination by first checking the woman for CRC (see discussion of the Organic Acid Test in Chapter 3) and the man in the equation for a low sperm or otherwise abnormal count. If she has a positive response to this test for Candida, he should be tested too! CRC can be a sexually transmitted disease, and can impair fertility. I have had several cases of infertility over the years, when the male partner had subclinical hypothyroidism (a subtle low-thyroid condition) and responded to T3 therapy with dramatic improvement in his sperm count, and a long-awaited baby!

QUESTION 7 Menstrual Disorders and Low Libido

All sorts of menstrual irregularity problems (premenstrual syndrome, irregular or absent periods, and so on) can be presenting signs of CRC. There is clearly an association between the complexities of the menstrual cycle and the symptoms of CRC. During certain parts of the menstrual cycle, estrogen hormone levels increase. The changing influence of estrogen alone, and estrogen plus progesterone together, reduces the ability of the vagina to inhibit the growth of the Candida.

The stressful emotional and behavioral swings of a woman's menstrual cycle can also impair sexual enjoyment and reduce sexual activity. Stress is both a result of CRC and a self-perpetuating cause. The initial stress response causes the release of adrenalin, a stress hormone, from the adrenal gland. Although adrenalin helps the body adapt to stress, it causes an instantaneous release of sugar from the liver store of glycogen. It also induces the release of cortisol (hydrocortisone), which produces a strong anti-inflammatory state throughout the body and a longer period of increased blood sugar levels. That combination fosters the growth of Candida.

QUESTION 8 Itch

Candida can be transferred between partners during oral sex (kissing mouth to mouth or mouth to genitals). It can be transmitted during genital sex and by sharing of towels, sheets, and generally careless contacts. Therefore, when the Candida organism is present in one partner, both partners should be treated simultaneously. While Sally and Richard each experienced itching in the genital or anal area, the itching may occur anywhere, with or without a rash, although constant scratching produces a rash. Sally was also taking birth control pills, which can cause an allergic reaction such as itching, and definitely changes the susceptibility of the vaginal lining to Candida.

QUESTION 9 Behavioral and Psychiatric Disorders

CRC is one of many chronic infections that can have a major impact on psychiatric disorders that are otherwise unexplainable, including behavior problems in children. Some years ago, Paul Fink, M.D., a former president of the American Psychiatric Association, suggested to fellow psychiatrists that anytime anyone who was previously healthy suddenly presented with any kind of psychiatric illness, the possibility that it was triggered by a chronic infection such as Lyme disease (caused by a bacterium known as *Borrelia burgdorferi*) should be considered. Unfortunately, Dr. Fink did not include CRC, the most common complication of the long-term antibiotics that are the mainstay of treatment for Lyme disease. Pediatric autoimmune neuropsychiatric disorder associated with *Streptococcus* (PANDAS), a condition that can cause a wide variety of nervous system symptoms, including irritability, extreme mood swings, hyperactivity, and problems with attention and concentration, is another example of a psychiatric diagnosis as a curable result of an infection treated with antibiotics. Unlike the treatment for ordinary strep throat, treatment of PANDAS frequently requires a much longer course of antibiotics, with two or more given either sequentially or simultaneously.

QUESTION 10 Hyperactivity

I see many hyperactive children. Hyperactivity is a primary characteristic of attention deficit hyperactivity disorder (ADHD), one of the most common mental disorders that develop in children.

When questioning parents of children who are hyperactive or have

ADHD, both of which cause a variety of learning and behavioral problems, they often report that their child was born with thrush or cradle cap and had infantile eczema, which was treated with steroids (cortisone derivatives) and topical antibiotics. Like oral antibiotics, topical antibiotics kill friendly bacteria, allowing pathogenic bacteria, viruses, and yeasts to take hold. These early health problems were often followed by respiratory allergies, starting with rhinitis (runny stuffy nose), otitis (ear infections) and/or asthmatic bronchitis (coughing and shortness of breath) that had been treated—not surprisingly—with oral antibiotics or steroids or both.

Is this somewhere in your child's past? When I hear that a child is born with thrush, as a physician treating CRC, I know that child was born with a yeast infection or Candida. What follows, if it is not treated at birth, are all of the health complications listed above—and more.

TEN TELLTALE BODY SIGNS

Do you relate to one of more of the maladies affecting my patients? If you do, and it has not been properly treated with diet, antifungal medications, and probiotics, I would highly suspect that you or your loved one has CRC. The following are ten telltale body signs you can check out at home that may confirm Candida has visited your body and moved in. This self-exam can be done in front of a mirror, but it is best to do it with a partner.

1. Do you have rough skin patches (can be rough and not be red.) in places where skin tends to be moist and droopy such as in skinfolds? Look at areas on your body that are not exposed to light or air. For example, many patients discover them under their breasts. These "rashes" have outside margins. Yet they form satellite lesions just outside the margins that spread until they coalesce; they will smell "yeasty."

2. Women, check to see if you have a vaginal secretion that is colorless or white. This discharge may have a yeasty odor but will not smell "fishy."

3. Look at your fingernails and toenails. Do the cuticles have redness at the bases?
4. Do you see a flaky dandruff (seborrhea) forming on your eyebrows and/or the hair on the back of your neck or scalp, or at the line connecting the outside of the nostril to the lip?
5. Do you have dandruff or severe eczema of the scalp?
6. Men, do you have jock itch or redness and itching in the perianal area? (If this is not Candida, you definitely have a fungal infection, so have it checked.)
7. Men, if you have not been circumcised, examine under the foreskin. Is there an itchy rash?
8. Look at your tongue. Is your tongue coated with white?
9. Do you have abnormally dry or oily skin?
10. Have you been losing your hair for no apparent reason?

All of these are signs you have Candida that has affected your skin, giving clear symptoms that your body is infected. Many of these skin signs are an allergic reaction to Candida in another place in your body! Pay attention to them. They will not get better without proper treatment, and I can promise they will get worse and cause more health problems without treatment.

3 Confirming It's CRC

Now I am going to give you the opportunity to get inside my head by telling you how I think when I make a diagnosis.

Unfortunately, diagnosing CRC is not as simple as getting a stool test or a blood workup. Because Candida is normally present in the mucous membranes of the mouth, intestines, and vagina, in both healthy and ill people, determining its presence doesn't confirm that it is thc source of a patient's health problems. Even if levels of Candida could be consistently and accurately counted in a laboratory setting, it may be impossible to know how tolerant one is to the Candida fungus and its toxic byproducts. People with strong immune systems may be capable of hosting large populations of Candida with a minimum of symptoms, while others, who are more sensitive, may feel a great deal of health stress as a result of mild Candida overgrowth. Then too it can be difficult to tell if Candida infection is a cause or a result of other illnesses—although Candida is almost always present when other intestinal, immune, or degenerative illnesses are present. Either way, reducing one's level of Candida will aid in healing.

Because of the challenging lifestyle-healing regimen that CRC recovery demands, most of us would like to have absolute confirmation of the diagnosis of Candida before embarking on (or continuing) a long and difficult CRC program. There are several available testing protocols for the Candida organism. Unfortunately, they all have limited accuracy. Even the most clinical of these is not able to decipher to what degree Candida is a problem for you, as an individual. Nonetheless, these tests are a valuable resource when part of an overall clinical assessment.

DIAGNOSTIC TOOLS AND TESTS

If from what you have read, you feel that Candida is a problem in your life or if you have been suffering with any of the disorders that I have been discussing as Candida related, I would like to help you get a proper diagnosis.

Not all doctors agree that Candida is important, or may consider it important in only the most extreme circumstances, but my experience has assured me that is not true. In the following section, I will tell you what to expect in the way of tests and treatments when you go to your doctor and ask to be tested for Candida, and I will tell you how I test for it. I hope that you will ask your doctor to include the tests that I do, and if she or he refuses, find a doctor who will do them so you can get an accurate diagnosis.

How Many Physicians Diagnose Candida

The following tests are the first ones most likely to be used to assess the presence of Candida.

1. Antibody testing: Antibodies are molecules that are made by the immune system to intercept or neutralize a specific invading organism or substance. This blood test can reveal whether your immune system has developed specific types of antibodies to "normal" or excess amounts of Candida. It will also tell the physician whether it's a past, active, or prolonged infection, depending on the level of the antibodies. If Candida is present, you need further testing. While high levels of IgA, IgG, and IgM antibodies to Candida can alert the physician to its presence, this test will not tell the physician if you have any other kind of sensitivity except that Candida exists in some way. The *absence* of anti-Candida antibod-

ies in a patient with definite Candida infection can be a major warning signal of severe immune incompetence.

2. Electrodermal testing: This diagnostic test evaluates the energetic pathways (acupuncture meridians) around the body's organs and systems with the use of a scanning instrument. Each acupuncture point on the skin's surface has a direct relationship to a specific organ and/or system in the body, by virtue of a characteristic energy field. Significant changes in these patterns from "normal" readings can indicate departures from optimum health. Electrodermal instruments have been programmed with the characteristic field patterns of hundreds of disease-causing microbes like Candida, and such patterns can therefore identify specific infections at various points in the body. The devices are also programmed to list results in order of seriousness to the body. Therefore, even if Candida was the original trigger, if the patient has a number of serious illnesses or consequential illnesses related to the Candida, the results for this test may be deceptively low as the other illnesses can overrun and mask the infection.

3. Medical history and symptom questionnaire: A detailed patient medical questionnaire helps to identify health symptoms and a history of Candida infection and antibiotic use.

4. Physical exam: A physical allows a doctor to examine the patient's body thoroughly. All the physician's sensory inputs may be involved. (Although tasting is rare nowadays, it was essential for centuries to detect sugar in the urine!) Many of the signs you checked yourself for in the previous chapter, a physician will look for as well. Flaky skin, seborrhea/dandruff, acne, eczema, psoriasis, a white-coated tongue, nail changes, inflammatory skin changes under skin folds, perianal rash, and vaginitis are strong visual clues that Candida may be present.

When the physical exam and medical history are completed, and the lab results are back, I discuss with the patient what is called the "differential diagnosis." This means that these are the different issues that might be causing the problem(s), and sometimes they're pretty far-fetched. When I note an unusual symptom or puzzling piece of information, I say to the patient: "One important thing I learned very early from a great diagnostician is, 'If you put your ear to the ground in the middle of the great plains of Kansas and you hear the distant thunder of hoof beats, you should think about horses—not zebras!'" Sure, I believe there are weird diagnoses, but they are few and far between. The physician should be focused on the most likely issues and test for them, first. It is true that there are some very serious maladies that also have to be considered, depending on the type of test that would be required, the expense and the logistics, and so on. They can be mentioned in passing and put off until later as more obvious diagnoses are ruled out.

My Basic Workup

At the same time that I'm gathering a patient's medical history and lab results, I am also performing my basic workup, which involves some or all of the following series of tests. These tests help me rule out coexisting medical problems. Each measures a particular set of markers that show how a specific organ of body system is functioning. Abnormal levels (either too low or too high; remember the Goldilocks principle?) can be significant, as imbalances can be present with a wide variety of acute and chronic illnesses. Ask your doctor to perform these tests.

1. Complete blood count (CBC) with differentials: A CBC calculates the composition and concentration of the basic cellular elements in the blood. A CBC measures the concentration of white blood cells (which fight infections), red blood cells (which transport oxygen), and platelets (which help with blood clotting) and aids in diagnosing conditions and disease such as infections, anemia, or blood cancers such as leukemia.

2. Basic metabolic panel (BMP): A BMP measures blood markers involved in the body's basic metabolic functions. At minimum, I test for the following: blood urea nitrogen (BUN) and creatinine

(two waste products normally filtered out of the blood by the kidneys); calcium (an important mineral needed for the release of hormones, transmission of chemical messages through the nerves, and muscular growth and contraction); glucose (a form of blood sugar that the body uses for energy and is controlled by the hormone insulin); and sodium, potassium, chloride, and carbon dioxide (electrolytes that help regulate body fluids and play a major role in regulating heart rhythm, muscle contraction, and brain function). Abnormal levels of these substances may be due to a variety of different medical conditions, including poor kidney function, hormone imbalances, diabetes or hypoglycemia (low blood sugar), and heart disease.

3. Liver function panel: Because the liver serves important functions in the body, including changing nutrients into energy for the body and breaking down toxic substances, I also check for blood levels of alkaline phosphatase (ALP); bilirubin; albumin, globulin, and total protein; uric acid; and at least two liver enzymes such as serum glutamic-oxaloacetic transaminase (SGOT) and serum glutamic-pyruvic transaminase (SGPT). Abnormal levels of any of these substances may indicate that liver damage or disease is present.

4. Thyroid function panel: These blood tests are used to evaluate the thyroid gland, which controls the speed of every metabolic reaction within the body all the way down to the cellular level. The panel measures thyroid-stimulating hormone (TSH); free thyroxine (T4); free triiodothyronine (T3); and the antithyroid antibodies, antithyroglobulin and antithyroid peroxidase. Abnormal levels can be a sign of thyroid disease, hypothyroidism (with symptoms such as fatigue, excessive weight gain, brain fog with memory loss), or hyperthyroidism (with opposite symptoms that can include weight loss, nervousness, tremor, increased heart rate, and insomnia).

5. Lipid panel: This blood test assesses the levels of fatty substances in a patient's blood. A lipid panel consists of measurements for total cholesterol; high-density lipoprotein (HDL, the so-called

good fraction thought to transport excess cholesterol out of the blood to the liver for disposal); low-density lipoprotein (LDL, the so-called bad fraction that transports cholesterol from the liver into the tissues and organs); and triglycerides (storage lipids that have a critical role in metabolism and energy production). High levels of total and LDL cholesterol, and triglycerides are a significant risk factor for heart disease.

Specific Tests I Use to Diagnose Candida

I like to have more objective monitors before determining that CRC is the source of a particular patient's health problem(s), so I perform three additional tests depending on how severe I believe the Candida to be and the results of the more preliminary testing.

1. Urine organic acid test: Organic acids are breakdown products that are produced from all the biochemical processes in the body (food digestion, cellular respiration, etc.) that keep it functioning. The body eliminates these waste products through the urine. The Organic Acids Test (OAT) from Great Plains Laboratory can detect up to seventy compounds found in the urine, from which amazingly accurate diagnostic impressions can be generated.

   Specifically, the test can check the organic acids a patient has in his or her urine that suggest the presence of a candida infection. Other markers indicate specific bacterial overgrowth, some beneficial and others disease-causing. The following substances are the ones I pay special attention to if I suspect a patient may have an overgrowth of Candida.

   - Arabinose: A toxic waste product released by yeast; an elevated level of arabinose in the urine signifies the presence of Candida yeast organisms growing in the body.
   - Tartaric acid: Another definitive diagnostic substance and toxic waste product released by the Candida; if elevated levels of tartaric acid (or arabinose) are found in an apparently healthy patient's urine, it is a definitive indicator of active colonization by Candida.

- Elevation of seven or eight other organic acids can further validate the presence of a Candida infection.

In addition, the OAT tests important metabolic functions in the rest of the body. Abnormal levels of certain organic acids can reveal the body's ability to absorb some vitamins and nutrients, metabolize fatty acids, produce and relay neurotransmitters (brain chemicals), burn its own fat (ketosis), and support the functioning of the Krebs cycle (a group of reactions that help turn food into energy). These measurements give the physician a wide range of information about a patient's overall health. The odds are very good that your mainstream doctor has not heard of this test. If she or he were to see patient results from the OAT, they would have no inkling of the useful information it provides! I have no official or financial ties to Great Plains Laboratory, or its director, William Shaw, Ph.D., but I believe he pioneered the use of this testing, which provides the most reliable results, with by far the most comprehensive explanation of abnormal values, as part of each report.

I believe that the OAT is a very important test for suspected but unconfirmed diagnosis of Candida when the patient does not have vaginitis (obviously that means all males), nor the symptoms of an irritable bowel with severe gas, distention, and bloating that so frequently accompanies a stool Candida invasion. Indeed, the reason this test is necessary is that in the worst cases, yeast organisms are frequently unable to be cultured from any body parts, because the yeast has been in the system so long that it has invaded the body and is no longer present in the stool or in the vagina. Most physicians believe this is evidence that there is no yeast infection. Unfortunately, as I've said, these patients can be the sickest and may have the worst problems, and in that situation the OAT can be a very rewarding inquiry. Tell your doctor that you want this test done.

2. Comprehensive stool analysis with anoscope exam: A comprehensive stool analysis is a series of tests used to determine which types of bacteria (beneficial, harmful, and disease-producing) are living in the intestinal tract and their levels. Some tests on stool can demonstrate incomplete digestion and inflammation from allergy

or infection or both, as well as evidence of gluten sensitivity. While stool analyses vary from lab to lab, a comprehensive test should always check for Candida. If Candida organisms are present, they are cultured to see if they will grow. If the unhealthy organisms are found, the good labs will test them to see which antibiotics or antifungal medications are most likely to be effective in eliminating them. I use several laboratories for stool analysis, including Doctor's Data, Genova Diagnostic, Great Plains Laboratories, and Diagnos-Techs, although the latter does not do drug resistance, or sensitivity, testing at the present time.

When the testing is done this way, and the body is positive for Candida, it is the very best way of making a diagnosis. If the test is negative, it does not mean that Candida is not present in the body. What it could mean is that the yeast has already penetrated the intestinal lining and is so deeply rooted in the body that it no longer is present as a colony in the stool. When the patient has all the signs of Candida, and the stool test is negative, then I perform a more advanced stool test. This test, called an anoscopy, is done by swabbing the lining of the rectum and submitting the sample to a laboratory to be cultured for yeast.

An anoscopy can be especially important for women who have had many vaginal yeast infections that suddenly stop recurring. When yeast does not show positive in the vagina, the doctor assumes there is not a yeast infection. This is one reason Candida infections are frequently overlooked by doctors—even those who have learned about Dr. Truss's finding that yeast problems start in the colon, but are not yet current with the latest discoveries about Candida and its diagnosis. When I began using this then new diagnostic test in 1985, I discovered the presence of the filamentous form (hyphae) of yeast as it was in the process of penetrating the mucosal lining, even in the absence of a positive stool culture. This insight I am proud to say was a major addition to the understanding of CRC. It helped explain to the various physicians (myself included), who for years had been puzzled by Dr. Truss's finding, how Candida could exist and escape detection by other testing methods.

I also discovered that in New York City, where I had a practice for years and performed many anscopies, more than 50 percent of the patients I tested for Candida had one or more parasites! That figure is probably higher than in many other areas of the country because of the high number of immigrants from poor countries who find work doing menial labor in restaurants and food stores such as fresh salad bars. Many come from countries where over 90 percent of the population are carriers of parasites, and have adapted to them, so that they have minimal symptoms, but traveler's diarrhea (also known as Montezuma's revenge and Trotsky's trots) are typical of the conditions that strike newcomers. This is an important reason why all employees who work with food must be instructed in their native language to wash their hands after using the lavatory.

Very few doctors perform anoscopies. If you feel this test is necessary for you, look for an infectious disease doctor in your area and call the office to make certain the doctor does it.

3. Skin, tissue, and secretion cultures: This lab test involves culturing various parts of the body—for example, in the moist folds of skin (under breasts or overhanging fat), in the groin, or between the buttocks, and from the walls of the bowel, vagina, sputum, nasal discharge, or tongue—to determine whether Candida can be demonstrated to grow. As is always true in suspected infections, a positive test is confirmative, but a negative test cannot prove the absence of an infection other than in the specimen that was tested.

4. Polymerase chain reaction (PCR) testing: It is now possible to identify the DNA of Candida from blood, stool, and urine specimens or from scraping from the tongue, tonsils, nose, ear, rectum, vagina, penis, skin folds and sores, and nails by PCR testing. One of its many benefits is that the test can detect and identify slow-growing bacterial infections at low levels within hours rather than weeks. I occasionally request a PCR test but again, while finding Candida is proof positive, not finding it means only that it is not in that specific specimen. It does not mean that Candida is not elsewhere in the body.

I know this sounds like a good deal of testing, and your head may be spinning from it. It is not any more complicated than having your doctor order the test you need for proper diagnosis. Keep in mind that your health comes first. You know better than anyone how you are feeling. Undiagnosed infections like Candida can sometimes be a major contributor to immune dysfunction, aging, and chronic degenerative diseases.

The chapter that follows may be another challenge for your doctor, because CRC must be treated vigilantly or it will not be under control. So take a deep breath and read on.

PART TWO

Treating Candida-Related Complex

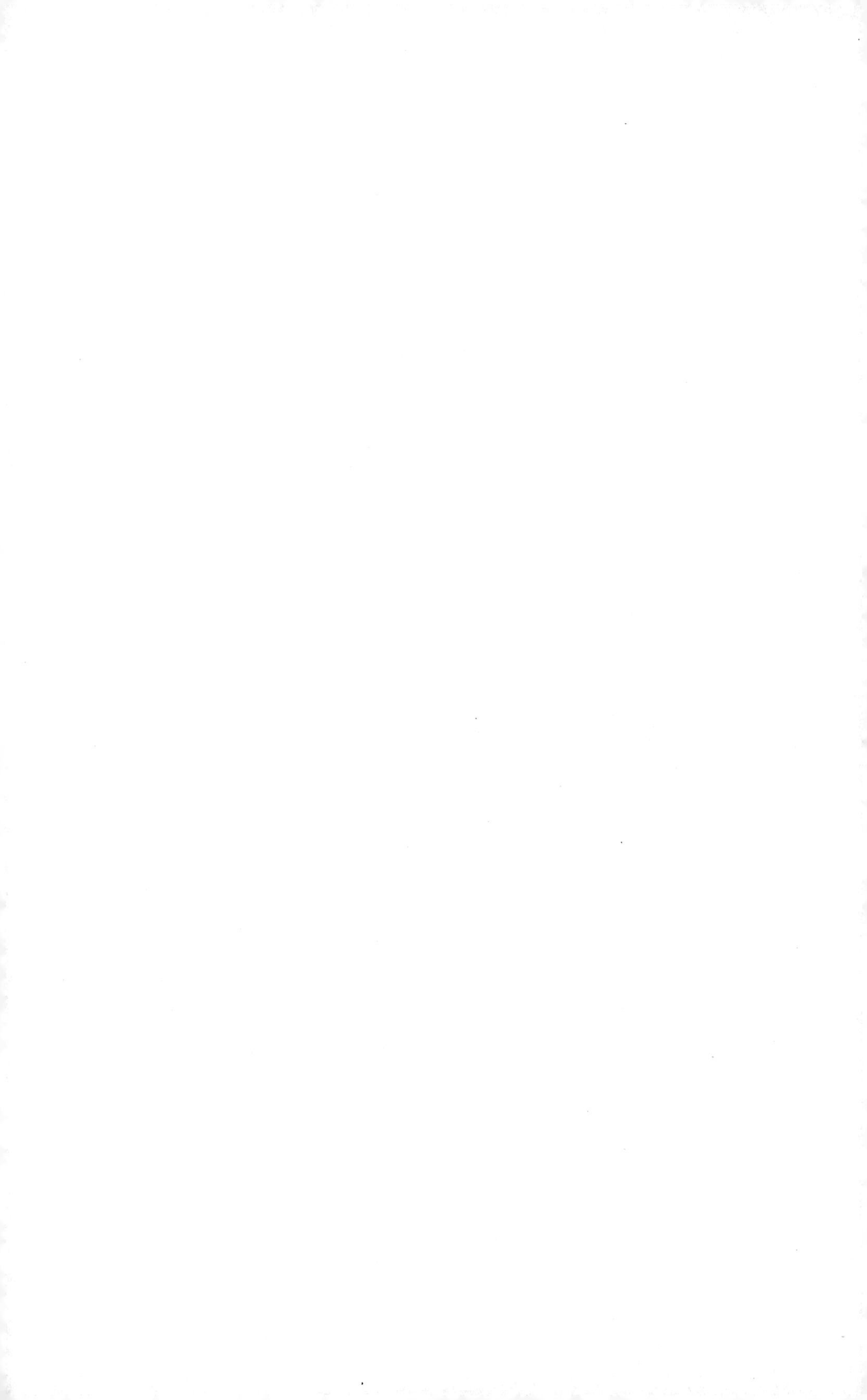

4 How I Treat CRC

Mainstream medicine has been brainwashed by the pharmaceutical industry into believing that prescription drugs are the answer to all disease, and that all a patient needs for recovery is one of their "magic pills." (Moreover, the newer the pill, the better.) It is as though the patient with his or her own unique body, mind, and spirit do not count in the healing process. It was this realization, you may remember, which led to my epiphany about integrative medicine and the inability to "fix" a patient by conventional medical means alone. What that means to me is that you as a patient and I as a physician cannot depend upon prescription drugs to do the body's work! To be sure, they are very important allies in the fight with Candida, but you must also step up to the plate and do your part!

In this chapter I attempt to explain the treatment options for CRC, both from a mainstream and integrative point of view. I achieve the best results when I combine all medical approaches, beginning with mainstream medicine and then adding complementary therapies. Once I'm convinced the diagnosis is CRC, I sit down with my patient and devise a treatment plan. My treatment evolves from all these therapeutic tools, and by correcting any immune deficiencies that have surfaced from the tests my patient took (discussed in the last chapter). The first priority in my treatment of Candida is the immune system, which lives mostly in the gut. When a person has digestive problems, the immune function is inhibited and cannot fight off infections—Candida or otherwise.

PRIORITY 1 BUILD A STRONG IMMUNE SYSTEM

Why treat the immune system? The presence of a Candida infection is always associated with some sort of immune difficulty. Your immune system is responsible for recognizing and identifying foreign substances in the body, and in some way or another initiates the process of utilizing or destroying the substances, then moving on. It doesn't matter if the initial infectious agent is a bacterium, virus, yeast, mold, fungus, or retrovirus (which is different from most viruses). When everything in the immune system is working perfectly, the body has a great head start toward being well balanced.

Your immune system sets up many barriers to keep toxins from entering the body. We, however, in our human (lack of) wisdom, bypass the barriers by eating, drinking, and breathing materials that are actually toxic—even though they are approved by the government's Food and Drug Administration (FDA). Think about it. We live in a way that's often contrary to non-toxic living. Most of us spend the majority of our time indoors, breathing in all the toxic materials we use to keep our homes "clean." We work in buildings whose windows don't open, so chemical-laden air is constantly recirculating. We eat foods that have been treated with pesticides and other chemicals. And when we finally have time for recreation, we go to a movie theater that has been sprayed with a chemical to make it smell good, or we jog in traffic, breathing in exhaust fumes. Removal of these toxins is essential to the restoring healthy functioning to a weakened immune system.

As I have said, the immune system is mostly in the gut; therefore to fight infections in general and CRC in particular, we must cleanse the gut first. Start by cleansing the accumulated toxins from your body with the following three-day detox. This detoxification method actually spans nine days: three to prepare for it, three to do the actual detoxification, and three to bring you to the point where you may begin a true Yeast-Free Diet. Keep in mind, that the first three to four days, you may feel much worse. This is an indication that toxins are being flushed out of your body. Once you are on the fifth day, you will begin feeling better.

Before beginning a detoxification, please consider the following:

- Your detoxification will be much more pleasurable if you think about it as doing something wonderful for your body.
- Concentrate on enjoying and nurturing yourself.
- Buy a natural-bristle brush with a long handle at your health food store. Brush your skin daily to release toxins. Toxins will be released through your skin and breath and excreted in your urine and feces.
- This is a perfect time to find a beach or a path in the woods where you can take a walk and breathe deeply, allowing your lungs to throw off toxins. Or at least practice yoga or gentle stretching in front of an air purifier or air-cleansing plant.
- Avoid heavy exercise.
- Try eating only organic foods. See if food begins to taste more flavorful, and you begin to feel really good.
- Read the detoxification instructions before beginning.
- Take the supplements recommended for detoxification support.
- Drink lots of water to wash away the toxins.
- Expect to urinate often for the first three to five days.
- If you are ill, over sixty-five, or more than forty pounds overweight, please consult your doctor before going on any detoxification program.

DAYS 1–3 Detox Preparation

Three days before starting this detoxification, take proteins out of your diet. Move toward vegetables and clear broth.

Prepare a light broth to use during your detoxification:

1 white onion, peeled and diced

10 garlic cloves, peeled

4 carrots, diced
2 stalks celery, diced
1 gallon of spring water
1 tablespoon sea salt or Herbamere (an herbal seasoning salt)

Place the vegetables and water in a saucepan. Bring to a boil. Reduce the heat and simmer for one hour. Strain the vegetables from the broth. Add at least one tablespoon of sea salt (more is okay, less is not). Salt will draw excess mucus into the intestines during a fast. Save the cooked vegetables you made the broth with for afterward.

EAT ORGANIC

The U.S. Department of Agriculture's revised organic standards, mandated by the new organic labeling law, will make it easy to tell if the food you are buying is organically produced. Today, organic seals appear on foods. A food is labeled as having one of the following:

- 100 percent organic ingredients
- 95–100 percent organic ingredients
- 50–95 percent organic ingredients

Labels that claim 50 percent organic ingredients may list specific organically produced ingredients on the information panel of the package, but may not make any organic claims on the front of the package.

DAYS 4–6 Detoxification Period

During these three days, you will eat fresh organic raw vegetables, drink juices made from fresh raw vegetables, and eat the broth made from bottled spring water and fresh vegetables, and seasoned with sea salt or Herbamere.

From morning to midday: Eat mostly raw vegetables (of your choice) and drink the salted broth. Take small bites and thoroughly chew your foods. Swallow what is in your mouth before taking another bite.

From midday to bedtime: Drink fresh vegetable juices home-squeezed from raw vegetables.

You may drink as much spring water as you wish throughout this three-day detoxification.

Relax during this detoxification. Meditate, rest or follow some of the suggestions in the bulleted list above. Brush your skin in the shower twice a day to remove toxins, and schedule a full body massage, if possible.

If you feel hungry, eat more vegetables or drink more broth.

DAYS 6–9 Toxin-Free and Ready to Go

Once you have completed the detox, this is the time to begin Dr. Levin's Yeast-Free Diet (discussed in Chapter 5).

DETOX SUPPLEMENT SUPPORT

Nutritional supplements are needed in greater amounts when the body is undergoing detoxification changes and can help make the detoxification process more efficient. Consider supplementing with the following nutrients:

- The herbals aloe vera (as the supplement MPS) to help cleanse the intestines, echinacea to boost the immune response, and rhodiola and ginseng to eliminate fatigue. (MPS, short for mucilaginous polysaccharides, is a glyconutrient produced in the body and also found in the gel of the aloe plant that is known to play a key role in immune system function.)
- Fiber supplements and herbal laxatives, which help flush out toxins and old fecal matter that may remain in the gastrointestinal tract.
- Digestants and enzymes of all kinds! Digestive supplements to help digest the fats, proteins, and carbohydrates in foods and reduce the stress on the digestive system. Look for a supplement that contains all the major enzyme groups—amylase, protease, and lipase.
- A liquid vitamin/mineral supplement such as IntraMax, which bonds carbon to your cells, detoxifying them, and then forcing the nutrients into the cell (1 ounce a day will do it).

- Essential fats and oils from krill and organic flaxseed, rich sources of omega-3 fatty acids, help to eliminate toxins and rebuild healthy cell membranes (take at least 1,000 international units daily).
- Immune modulators are antioxidants that are important in detoxification. They are present in IntraMax (see above); add also three packets a day of lipospheric vitamin C to help avoid withdrawal symptoms during detox.

All these supplements are available at your local health food store or online.

PRIORITY 2 STOP FEEDING THE CANDIDA

Your vegetable detox will be a helpful transition as you begin to cut out foods that the Candida organism loves and encourages its growth.

The Sugar and Yeast Families of Foods

Candida thrives on sugar—any form of sugar. This includes natural sugars and artificial sweeteners, alcohol, and simple carbohydrates (like white bread, pasta, and other processed foods). These all cause a rapid rise in blood sugar and feed all yeasts, including Candida. Yeast also grows best when it is fed sugar (think of rising bread). Likewise, eating foods that contain yeast cause the foods to ferment in the gut and feed the Candida. This includes all products baked with yeast such as bread, cookies, cakes, and all foods that form yeast as they age or dry such as molded cheeses, many nuts that have not been refrigerated, and dried herbs. Foods that are fermented in a yeast culture such as vinegars, wine, beer, and most alcohol are considered part of the yeast family of foods and are also to be avoided.

PRIORITY 3 TAKE SOMETHING TO *KILL* THE CANDIDA

There are many different types of antifungal products and medications. Many herbs are natural antifungal agents. Increasing your intake of them either in foods or supplements will help fight the Candida infection, so I recommend them to all my patients. When necessary, effective but strong prescription antifungal medication can also be called upon.

Natural Antifungals

Natural antifungals for yeast infections are easy to find. They can be found in larger grocery stores and in health food stores, or can be ordered online.

- Garlic: This herb contains a large number of compounds that exhibit potent antifungal properties, including allicin, alliin, and allinase. Eat lots of it or try taking it in capsule form.
- Grapefruit seed extract: Also known as citrus seed extract, this powerful Candida-killer comes from the pulp and seeds of grapefruit. Strong tasting, the extract is available as a liquid concentrate or in tablets.
- Oregano oil: A potent antiviral, antibacterial, and anti-inflammatory, powerful in killing a range of fungi. *Oregano vulgare,* as opposed to *Oregano marjoram* (a seasoning in Italian food), is usually supplied as an oil in supplement form.
- Monolaurin: This long-chain fatty acid found in coconut oil not only damages the Candida organism but also helps restore the stomach to its correct acidity. Monolaurin is available in supplements or from eating coconut oil.
- Tannins: A group of compounds called polyphenols that are found in the seeds and stems of grapes, the bark of some trees, and tea leaves. Because of their sharp, bitter taste, tannins are easiest to take in a supplement such as Tanalbit.

Prescription Antifungals

There are numerous Candida-killing medications available. All of them are meant to target yeast overgrowth—some at specific stages and in different areas in or on the body. Make certain your doctor gives you specific instructions on how to take any of the prescription antifungal drugs listed below. Many of them have side effects, including interactions with other medications.

- Oral non-absorbable antifungal drugs: Because these drugs are not absorbed from the intestinal tract, they work best for early stage local Candida infections that have not taken root (become systemic) in the body. They are generally used for treating yeast infections of the intestinal tract, vagina, mouth, and skin such as athlete's foot, jock itch, and ringworm, and include nystatin, Ancobon (flucytosine), Fungizone/Amphocin (amphotericin B), and Mycelex Troche (clotrimazole).
- Oral absorbable antifungal drugs: These medications are generally prescribed for later stage systemic yeast infections that have taken root and spread to organs and different parts of the body through the bloodstream. These antifungals are absorbed from the intestines and into the bloodstream. The most effective agents in this group are the conazole-based medications, which include Diflucan (fluconazole), Noxafil (posaconazole), Nizoral (ketoconazole), Sporanox (itraconazole), and Vfend (voriconazole).
- Topical antifungal agents: These preparations are used for superficial skin, hair, and nail infections such as athlete's foot, jock itch, and many (unrecognized) diaper rashes that are severe and unresponsive to baby lotions and creams, and include Lamisil (terbinafine), Lotrimin (clotrimazole), Desenex (miconazole), and a host of over-the-counter vaginal creams, douches, and ointments.
- Intravenous antifungal drugs: Echinocandins are the first class of injectable antifungal drugs used to treat local and systemic Candida infections. They include Cancidas (caspofungin), Eraxis (anidulafungin), and Mycamine (micafungin).

PRIORITY 4 TAKE PROBIOTICS

Probiotic supplements reintroduce colonies of helpful or beneficial bacteria to the intestinal tract. They not only help crowd out the Candida yeast, but they also repopulate the gut tract with healthy intestinal bacteria, which boosts the immune system and helps maintain the correct levels of acidity in the stomach.

Most probiotic supplements are a combination of several species of bacteria. The most common are *Lactobacillus acidophilus, Bifidobacteria bifidum,* and *Eschericia coli,* with various strains of each. Every strain is different. (Think of influenza with its Hong Kong flu, swine flu, avian flu, Asian flu; they all cause the flu, but they are different.) The more variety of beneficial bacteria you put into your digestive tract, and the greater the number of colony-forming units (CFUs), the harder it is for the unhealthy bacteria to survive.

It is important to change brands every two months to obtain a maximum mixture of healthy bacteria. Some people take different brands every day or two. While that's the right idea, I think it's too short a time to get these new flora to push their way in. Changing products every six to eight weeks provides a better chance for each strain to set up housekeeping, and I believe that if it hasn't taken root by then, it probably isn't going to this time.

Some probiotic products contain prebiotics, non-digestible foods that feed the probiotics. Prebiotics act like fertilizer for the probiotics. They help to soothe and heal the intestinal tract as well as provide much needed fiber to help get rid of toxins.

PRIORITY 5 AVOID THE MAJOR CRC TRIGGERS

Avoid a high sugar diet and the unnecessary use of antibiotics, steroid drugs, birth control pills, and stomach acid suppressants. Seek out other alternatives. All upset the balance of bacteria in the gastrointestinal tract and weaken the immune system, making your body more susceptible to the proliferation of Candida.

PRIORITY 6 FOLLOW A YEAST-FREE DIET

In the next chapter, I will describe the three progressive phases of my Yeast-Free Diet, which focuses on helping to strengthen immune defense, kill off yeast, and restore healthy bacteria, so your body is able to control abnormal growth of Candida on its own and help keep it in check over the long run.

EVERY TREATMENT PROGRAM HAS RISKS

Whenever possible, natural therapies such as nutritional and herbal supplements, probiotics, and diet along with natural antifungals are recommended. However, in some cases, these measures are not enough and stronger prescription medications are needed. Keep in mind that every treatment program has risks. Believe it or not, I've even heard of problems resulting from taking probiotics!

If your recovery involves prescription medication, the most important issues that should be checked regularly (every two to four weeks) are the body's complete blood count with differentials (page 26) and the liver function panel (page 27). All prescription antifungal conazole-based drugs (page 42) can adversely affect the blood and metabolic liver enzymes, and minor abnormalities need to be rechecked more often. Each practitioner has his or her own "worry level." For instance, the two most common changes in liver tests are increasing SGPT and SGOT enzyme levels (abnormal levels may indicate liver damage.) Liver specialists are so accustomed to seeing high levels that they have a greater tolerance for small changes (above the reference range), whereas your doctor may not. For everyone's peace of mind, encourage your doctor to carefully monitor your blood workups.

Another common side effect of taking any of the absorbable antifungals is an aggravation of previously existing Candida symptoms. This reaction is called a "die-off" (or Herxheimer reaction) and occurs when yeast cells are rapidly killed. This tends to occur much less frequently in individuals who are taking only natural antifungals. These symptoms normally clear up in a week or shortly thereafter, and you should soon be feeling better.

5 Dr. Levin's Yeast-Free Diet

with Fran Gare, N.D.

Dr. Levin's Yeast-Free Diet is your companion to the vitamins, nutrients, probiotics, herbal yeast inhibitors, and antifungal drugs (if you are taking them) used to treat CRC. All of these nutritional measures and therapies together will bring you back on the path to a healthy immune response. The diet is perhaps the most challenging of the treatments because it encompasses your daily lifestyle. However, with each of its three progressive phases of eating, it becomes easier, and you may enjoy it as you begin to feel healthier and more energized. Each phase lasts approximately one month.

BASIC GUIDELINES FOR GOING YEAST-FREE

The object of Dr. Levin's Yeast-Free Diet is to eliminate foods that contain sugar and feed the Candida yeast, as well as foods that contain yeasts and molds that promote yeast growth. In general, the following guidelines apply to all three phases of Dr. Levin's Yeast-Free Diet. These foods are to be avoided, except when noted in each phase.

Foods to Eliminate

- **Sugar, chocolate, and sweets.** This includes any and all forms of sugar, including white and brown sugars; honey and molasses; barley malt, corn syrup, maple sugar or syrup, rice syrup; dextrose, fructose, glucose, maltose, and sucrose; artificial sweeteners; and foods containing these sugars such as sodas and candy. Read food labels to make your food does not contain hidden sugars. Try xylitol instead.

- All types of **alcoholic beverages** such as beer, wine, and distilled liquor like whiskey, gin, rum, and vodka are high in sugar and are fermented liquids. Yeast is used to ferment foods.
- **Fresh fruit, dried fruit,** and **fruit juices.** Sugar is sugar, and even the natural sugars in fruit encourage the growth of yeasts; the skins of fruits and melons (especially cantaloupe) accumulate mold during growth. Fruit juices (bottled, canned, and frozen), as well as canned tomatoes and tomato juice, contain citric acid, a common preservative that promotes yeast growth. One exception: Fresh lemon juice is low in sugar and improves the taste of food, so small amounts may be used throughout the diet.
- **Milk** (whole, skim, and fat-free), and all **dairy products** and **cheeses**. Avoid buttermilk, cream, ice cream, sour cream, kefir and yogurt, as well all cheeses, including cottage cheese. Milk contains lactose (milk sugar) and cheeses of all kinds, especially aged cheeses and moldy cheeses like Roquefort, contain yeasts and/or fungi. Clarified butter (ghee) or butter (in moderation) may be used.
- Commercial **baked goods**, including breads, biscuits, buns, rolls, pretzels, crackers, and pastries are quickly converted into sugar; most baked goods are also made with baker's yeast.
- **Wheat, barley, rye, semolina, spelt, and oats** are carbohydrates that convert to sugars during digestion.
- **Starchy vegetables** (beets, carrots, corn, green peas, potatoes, sweet potatoes, yams, and all winter squash) cause a rapid rise in blood sugar levels.
- **Fungi** of all kinds, including mushrooms, truffles, and morels, are relatives of yeast.

- Raw and roasted **nuts** accumulate mold and must be temporarily omitted.
- All **fermented condiments, sauces, and vinegar-containing foods** should be avoided. Prepared mayonnaise, mustard, ketchup, barbecue sauce, soy sauce, tamari; pickled vegetables, sauerkraut, horseradish, relishes, green olives, and commercial salad dressing; and vinegar and vinegar-containing salad dressings fall into this category. Vinegar-free dressings and mayonnaise can be substituted.
- Molds build up on **pickled, smoked,** and **dried meats, fish,** and **poultry,** including bacon, ham, sausages, salami, hot dogs, luncheon meats, pickled tongue, corned beef, pastrami, smoked sardines, and other processed meat and fish during processing and should not be eaten.
- Drinks, cereals, and candies to which **malt** has been added should be avoided.
- **Tea, coffee, spices,** and **dried herbs** can easily become contaminated with mold. Cinnamon, an antimicrobial, can be used. Fresh herbs may be used and frozen for future use.
- Throw out all **leftover food** if not consumed (or frozen) within twenty-four hours. Molds grow quickly on leftovers.
- Many **medications** and **nutritional supplements** are derived from yeasts or molds and should be avoided. Herbal tinctures containing alcohol should also be temporarily eliminated. Check labels and look for preparations that specify they are yeast-free and alcohol-free.

You may think of what you are about to read as restricting your lifestyle. The only way for you to find out how healthy you will feel when following the diet is to do it.

Phase 1 is the most rigorous stage of the diet. It requires going "cold carbs," as it restricts all carbohydrates. For those of you who have "done" Atkins to lose weight, you "get" it. For those who have not been on a carbohydrate-restricted diet in the past, please read Phase 1 of the diet carefully, and go shopping for food before you begin.

When you begin Phases 2 and 3, you will feel rewarded, as you can add many of your favorite foods back into your diet. I want you to understand all you can about the foods you are eating, so the following is Nutrition 101 just for you.

NUTRITION 101

Carbohydrates, proteins, and fats are the three basic building blocks of which food is made.

Carbohydrates

There are two kinds of carbohydrates: simple and complex.

Simple carbohydrates are sugars and starches that are digested mostly in your mouth and esophagus (that is, before they reach your stomach) by an enzyme called salivary amylase. Examples of simple carbohydrates are commercial white, pumpernickel, rye, and whole-wheat breads, pasta, cakes, and cookies (and any product with a first, second, or third ingredient listed on the label as white or enriched white flour). All simple sugars, including corn syrup, rice syrup, barley malt, molasses, honey, maple sugar or syrup, beet sugar, dextrose, sucrose, fructose, glucose, maltose (almost anything that ends with *-ose*) are simple carbohydrates. Fruit and some starchy vegetables such as potatoes, beets, green peas, and carrots contain simple sugars and have to be regulated while you are on Dr. Levin's Yeast-Free Diet. These foods easily ferment in your gut causing an overgrowth of yeast.

Digestion of complex carbohydrates begins in the mouth, but then continues through the digestive system in many steps, until these carbohydrates arrive in the small intestine. There, an enzyme called alpha-amylase, excreted by the pancreas, eventually converts the complex carbohydrates to simple sugars. This is a slower process. Many complex carbohydrates are added back into your diet in Phases 2 and 3.

Complex carbohydrates include all grains (amaranth, barley, couscous, kasha [buckwheat], millet, oats, orzo, quinoa, rice, spelt, wheat), most dried beans, some starchy vegetables, and even green vegetables. Because complex carbohydrates convert to simple sugars, they cause a slow rise in blood sugar levels.

Proteins

Dr. Levin's Yeast-Free Diet is high in meat or fish protein, eggs (a complete source of life—chickens are hatched from them), and a small amount of dairy (cheese is added in Phase 3). If you are a vegan or believe that a macrobiotic diet is the only way to eat, you will find this yeast-free diet very challenging. However, if you are approaching forty, are a vegan, and find that you have CRC, and your body is unexpectedly changing in a way that makes you unhappy, please open your mind to what I have to say. It could change your life.

Proteins are a combination of twenty-two amino acids, eight of which are essential to life and cannot be made by your body.

Proteins form the framework of every cell in your body. About 50,000 proteins are used by the body in the formation of your muscles, hormones, and nerves. As we age, firm, well-formed muscles, balanced hormones, and steady nerves are key. Your body has an enzyme system made from proteins that is responsible for the normal functioning of your organs. The antibodies that protect you from illnesses are proteins, and unless your body has a high-quality source of the eight essential amino acids (these eight can usually make the fourteen others), your body cannot use any of them. Animal protein is our only source of complete protein. Proteins from vegetables, beans, and grains are incomplete because they lack one or more essential amino acids.

Your body has to work harder to burn and metabolize a protein than to burn and metabolize a carbohydrate or fat. For example, when you eat 100 protein calories, 30 of the 100 calories are used to metabolize the protein.

You have learned from this book that Candida can have a deleterious effect on the thyroid gland. A diet rich in essential amino acids (proteins) helps your thyroid gland convert T4 thyroid hormone into T3 thyroid hormone. T3 regulates the metabolism of most nutrients: the more available T3, the more efficient your metabolism. And, the big payoff when dieting yeast-free is that proteins do not promote the proliferation of Candida.

Fats

Fats are not restricted on Dr. Levin's Yeast-Free Diet. However, we do suggest that you eat only healthy fats. Here are great everyday reasons why you can eat healthy fats. Because they are healthy, taste wonderful, are yeast-free, and . . .

- Your brain cannot function without healthy fats because it is composed of 60 percent fat.
- Your sex hormones are manufactured from fat.
- When there is no fat under your skin, you wrinkle more easily.
- Healthy fats are more filling. You will eat less.
- Lack of healthy fats causes alligator skin, unmanageable hair (even hair loss), and cracked and split nails.
- Healthy fats have fewer calories than the fats in processed foods. When you eat them in moderation, your body metabolizes them as energy instead of as fatty deposits.
- Healthy fats reduce inflammation.

The most important fats to include in your diet come from fish, nuts, seeds, and some vegetables, and contain essential fatty acids. (Fats are actually fatty acids—that is, they consist of one fat molecule and one acid molecule.) These fatty acids are called "essential" because they are necessary for everyday body functions, and your body cannot make them. In fact, you cannot live without them. So you must either consume them as part of your diet or take them as nutritional supplements. These oils can be monounsaturated or polyunsaturated. They are liquid at room temperature.

Modern food processing has tampered with these health-giving oils, heating and refining them, exposing them to light and oxygen. As a result, the oil products on your grocer's shelves are rancid even before you open the bottle. Rancid oils are called lipid peroxides (or damaged fatty acids). When you eat them they use up the antioxidants in your liver, robbing your body of vitamins E and C. Rancid oils can cause every cell of your body that they come in contact with to become rancid. Monounsaturated and polyunsaturated vegetable, nut, and seed oils contain essential fatty acids of the omega-6 group. To stay fresh, they must be packaged in black glass or dark brown plastic and kept in a cool place on the shelves of your supermarket or health food store. They should be labeled "cold pressed" and have a seal under the cap. Please refrigerate all oils after opening them, even though the bottles do not instruct you to do so.

Another important oil to consume is fish oil, a polyunsaturated fat. Fish oils are a rich source of omega-3 fatty acids. They taste best eaten as fish (preferably wild fish). Fish oils are essential to glowing good health, so if you are not eating fatty fish like salmon, sardines, mackerel, trout and herring at least three times a week, you may want to take omega-3 fatty acid nutritional supplements.

Other important oils to include in your diet come from saturated sources of fats. Saturated fats tend to be semi-solid or solid at room temperature. Saturated fat is found in animal fats and tropical oils such as coconut and palm oils. Saturated fats have gotten a bad rap of late. But these saturated fats are not the dangerous synthetically hydrogenated types, which have received so much attention for their effect on health. Saturated fats play many important roles in your body. They are immune enhancers, are necessary for healthy bones, provide energy and structural integrity to your cells, and protect your liver. In addition, saturated fats enhance your body's use of essential fatty acids, do not use its antioxidant reserve, and are the only source of vitamins A, B_{12} and D.

Certainly eating non-organic animal fats is unhealthy. When you do eat animal fats they should be organic, and free of growth hormones and antibiotics.

For a list of which oils to buy and why, see the inset on page 52.

WHICH OILS TO BUY?

In my experience the following oils, when carefully selected and used as suggested, are the most healthy to consume and cook with. Each has its own antioxidant protection and is least likely to become rancid.

- **Extra-virgin olive oil** is the oil of choice for everyday use. It is the most versatile oil. Because it naturally contains vitamin E (an antioxidant that protects it from becoming rancid), it can safely be heated for sautéing* to a temperature of 325°F. If you are daring and love strong flavors, add fresh garlic or chilies to the bottle before refrigerating.
- **Macadamia nut oil** is 85 percent monounsaturated oil with a high smoke point and can be stored at room temperature for up to two years. I recommend sautéing and stir frying with it. It will remain stable (not hydrogenate) up to 410°F. I use it for most everything because of its light delicious taste.
- **Sesame oil** is my favorite to use with fish. I love to rub it on the fish before I poach or sauté it. It adds great flavor to other foods, too. Try it on vegetables or in your favorite salad dressing. Sesame oil contains a naturally occurring antioxidant, sesamol, which protects it from becoming rancid. You can sauté with sesame oil at 325°F. Although sesame oil is sometimes used for stir-frying, I do not recommend that you heat it that hot.
- **Walnut oil** has a great nutty flavor. You can use it for sautéing to 325°F, or anywhere you wish to add a nutty flavor.
- **Linseed (flax) and hemp oils** are other very important oils in this category. Linseed oil comes from the seeds of the flax plant and hemp oil from the seeds of the hemp plant. They are two of the most nutritious oils available. They are rich sources of alpha-linolenic acid, the precursor to omega-3 fatty acids sources. Because these oils turn rancid easily, they are very fragile and require special care. They also cannot be heated to high temperatures without losing their health benefits. For this reason, they are best used in salad dressings.
- **Coconut oil/butter** is a naturally saturated vegetable product. It is a type of fat called a medium-chain triglyceride, or MCT. MCTs metabolize more efficiently then other fats. They convert into energy instead of fat. Coconut

butter is an MCT and contains the powerful antioxidant lauric acid, also known as monolaurin, which is also an antifungal (used to treat viruses as lethal as HIV). It is the only fat I recommend for frying or baking at high temperatures. Coconut butter is tasty and can be used in all your food preparation. However, you *must* use it to fry or bake. It is the only healthy vegetable oil that does not become rancid, and will not hydrogenate and become a trans fat when heated to high temperatures. This oil is solid at room temperature (up to 76°F) and liquid at body temperature.

- **Red palm oil** is made from the fruit of the palm tree and contains about 50 percent naturally saturated fats and 50 percent unsaturated fats (predominately monounsaturated). Red palm oil's high level of antioxidants keeps it semi-solid at room temperature. It can be used for frying when you prefer not to have a slight coconut taste to your food.
- **Clarified organic butter** (butter with the milk solids removed) works well for sautéing at temperatures that do not exceed 350°F. You can buy clarified butter in health food or gourmet stores. It should be organic to avoid the antibiotics and growth hormones injected into non-organic cows. You can also make it yourself (for the recipe see page 66). Clarified butter, also known as ghee, is liquid at body temperature and is preferable to butter, especially for those who have milk sensitivities.

* Note: Sautéing is done at a lower temperature than stir-frying. If water sizzles when you drop it into fat that means the fat is hotter than 350°F, which is too hot for any oil other than macadamia, palm, or coconut oils. You may need to use a thermometer at first to learn how to judge the temperature of your oil.

Now that you know why you will be eating the foods on Dr. Levin's Yeast Free Diet, let's look at the diet.

PHASE 1

Phase 1 eliminates most sources of sugar and yeast from your diet. Although restrictive, it is healthy and important to your success. The foods you can eat consist of the following proteins and fats. Carbohydrates are to be avoided during this phase.

- Quality protein at every meal, including: wild seafood and fish, free-range poultry and fowl, and grass-fed meats.
- A wide variety of fresh vegetables, raw or cooked, preferably organic.
- Cold-pressed nut, seed, and vegetables oils.
- Spring or filtered water daily with several squirts of lemon if you like. Avoid tap water, which may be contaminated with bacteria or parasites.

Remain on Phase 1 for approximately four weeks. There is not a limit to the amount of food that you can eat. Your appetite will self-regulate after the fifth day on the diet. It is important not to go off of the diet. If you feel hungry, eat as much as you wish of the foods allowed on the diet. Protein foods are best. If in question about what you can and cannot eat, refer back to the Guidelines for Going Yeast-Free on pages 45–47. The recipes and meal suggestions found in the next chapter will help start you on your way.

PHASE 2

As you move on to Phase 2 of your diet, you are able to enjoy more of a variety of foods. Raw, vacuum-packed, and unshelled nuts and seeds, raw nut butters, and beans are added along with some dairy (cream cheese, fresh chèvre, farmer's cheese, feta, Mexican queso fresco, mozzarella, and ricotta), preferably from goat or sheep milk, which give you a chance to enjoy much more tasty dishes. Beverages suitable to add during this phase are bancha and pau d'arco teas; these herbal teas are powerful antifungal agents.

PHASE 3

In Phase 3 you can add three ounces of semi-hard cheeses like Swiss, Cheddar, and Gouda a day, heavy cream, plain yogurt, and some complex carbohydrates in half-cup portions. Try organic brown rice, wild rice, and quinoa, and see if any of your symptoms return. You may also add small quantities of starchy vegetables (if no adverse reaction occurs) and low-carbohydrate fruits in half-cup serving (see listing of fruits below).

Fresh fruits are a fine source of vitamins, minerals, and fiber. They are also an excellent replacement for highly refined carbohydrate foods such as candy, cookies, and cakes. You may select any three from the "A" or "B" lists below per day, or two from the "C" list. Example: one small avocado, one-half cup of fruit salad, and one-half cup of honeydew melon, or one small orange and two slices of pineapple. The "A" list is best, of course. Avocados are the most beneficial of the fruits, so if you like them, make certain to include them in your diet.

Note: Bananas contain 23 percent carbohydrate and are not permitted. All fruits must be fresh. Fruits frozen or dried (raisins, apricots, etc.) or packed in a syrup are absolutely forbidden. Fruit juices are not permitted as a beverage. Home-squeezed vegetable juices are now permitted.

A List: 7 % Carbohydrate

Avocado—1 small

Rhubarb—1/2 cup

B List: 10% Carbohydrate

Blueberries—1/2 cup

Cantaloupe—1/2 cup

Casaba melon—1/2 cup

Coconut (fresh only)—1/4 cup

Honeydew melon—1/2 cup

Lemon—juice of 2 (fresh only)

Muskmelon—1/2 cup

Strawberries—1/2 cup

C List: 15% Carbohydrate

Apple—1 small

Apricot—1 small

Blackberries—1/2 cup

Loganberries—1/2 cup

Peach—1 small

Plum—1 average size

Cherries—$^{1}/_{2}$ cup

Dewberries—$^{1}/_{2}$ cup

Elderberries—$^{1}/_{2}$ cup

Grapefruit—$^{1}/_{2}$ large

Orange—1 or $^{1}/_{2}$ cup

Raspberries—$^{1}/_{2}$ cup

Pineapple—2 slices

Tangerine—1 average size

Youngberries—$^{1}/_{2}$ cup

TRANSITION

After you have completed the three phases of the diet, make sure you are retested for Candida. If you are Candida-free, you can carefully begin to add more whole grains, multiple servings of fruit and starchy vegetables, and a small amount of alcohol (vodka or aquavit is preferred) into your diet. One glass of red wine with a high protein meal is fine in most cases. You will always want to avoid sugary foods and other simple carbohydrates (most things white in color) to help keep your Candida overgrowth from ever returning again.

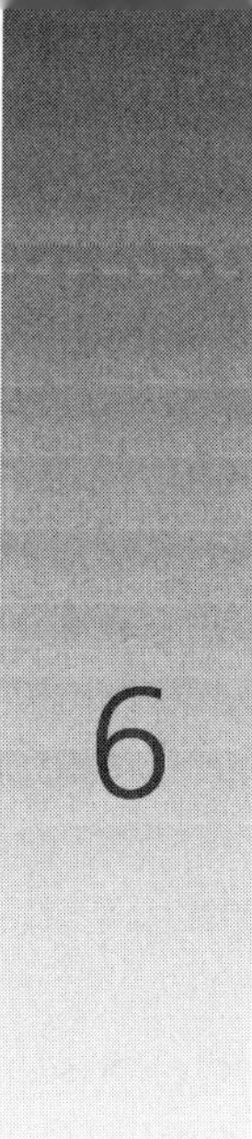

6 Recipes and Meal Plans

with Fran Gare, N.D.

Now that you know what your beginning food choices are, how about joining me in a "virtual trip" to your supermarket? I would like you to take that trip with me now. It will get you started on your diet program even before you begin the diet preparation. The only requirement is that you make your choices among the foods I mention here. They are all foods you can eat on the three phases of your diet. Each recipe is marked with the proper phase or phases. Please choose a supermarket that stocks certified organic foods. It's important that you eat the cleanest foods, free of pesticides, chemicals, waxes, and dyes.

LET'S GO SHOPPING

On all three phases of the diet, meat is a healthy protein and should be eaten and enjoyed. Meat from free-range (grass-fed) animals is best.

Poultry

Chicken, turkey, and duck are healthy eating on all three phases of your Yeast-Free Diet plan. Poultry including eggs should always be organic.

Fish

I hope your market has fresh wild-caught fish. We'll make that counter our next stop. Unless you are allergic to fish, I hope you'll choose several that you like, and I'll help you prepare them in the most delicious ways. Most of my fish recipes include oil as one ingredient, so let's look next at the oils.

Fats and Oils

Once again, all oils should be organic. Oils turn rancid when exposed to air and light. To avoid this, add one 400 international units (IU) capsule of vitamin E and an one-quarter teaspoon of powdered vitamin C to each bottle of oil that you open. Then refrigerate it. I would choose some extra-virgin olive oil packaged in a dark bottle, walnut oil, organic flax (linseed oil), hemp oil, sesame oil (especially good with fish), and red palm, macadamia, and coconut oils. I love these added to vegetables and in salad dressings. Try using them for light low-temperature sautéing, too. When you bake and fry, please choose clarified butter (ghee) and coconut oil. Butter (if tolerated) is permissible in minimal amounts when clarified butter is not an option (for example, in some restaurants).

Fresh Produce

Next, we'll look at the fresh produce. Isn't it inviting? Here we can choose among broccoli, asparagus, string beans, spinach, onions, garlic, celery, cucumber, scallions, and a few types of lettuces. These will make a fresh, flavorful salad. Stop by the *fresh* herbs. Look at the Seasoning Mixes in the recipe section and choose some you will enjoy eating. They will add great variety to your meals and make them much more flavorful. Remember, most of us have grown up using dried herbs and herbs from shakers. You will not be using them on this eating plan. They collect mold as they dry. Use fresh or frozen herbs only.

On Phases 1 and 2, your snacks will be pure protein. On Phase 3, you will begin enjoying fruits, so shop accordingly. Now we need some things for snacking. When fruit shopping, buy small amounts of two varieties of fruit. Choose from blueberries, plums, apricots, or grapefruit.

These foods are keys that open the door to a healthier, yeast-free body that will look and function the way you remember it did. With your cart piled high with fresh, nutritious foods, don't you feel better already?

Now that we have shopped together, step into my kitchen.

LET'S GET COOKING

These recipes challenge the taste buds. You may find some old favorites among them, but don't be surprised if they taste subtly different—more interesting, a little more sophisticated, healthier. I believe food should be as healthful as it tastes, and in this case be free of yeast. I hope you find these recipes to be full of delicious surprises. They can also be used on gluten-free and low carbohydrate diets. Not only you, but also all you cook for can lose weight and get healthier eating your food.

I hope you will take the time to make the broths, and freeze them for later use in the recipes. The broths add so much rich flavor.

Next, look at the herbal seasonings and see if there are any you may want to use often. Purchase the herbs and mix them in a three-ounce shaker bottle, and freeze what you don't use.

Everything you need to complete each recipe is listed at the top of each page. Cooking is far more enjoyable when the necessary ingredients for a recipe are at your fingertips. Take the time to assemble all of them before beginning to cook. Then your cooking experience will be fun, and you will feel relaxed and proud of what you have created. Eating the finished product will be a joyful gastronomic experience.

You may cut the recipes down if the portions are more than you and your family need, or you can freeze the extra amounts for another time. When yeast-free dieting, it is always good to have tasty meals that can be quickly defrosted to quench a sudden hunger, to avoid boredom ("not broiled chicken, again!"), or for those evenings when you arrive home tired and fantasize that the cook will have dinner on the table.

And don't forget guests. There isn't a guest who wouldn't leave the table with a smile on her or his face after a dinner cooked from these recipes. So you decide if you want to make a full recipe or cut it in half. You will feel like a talented cook either way.

A few words about our preference for several ingredients used in the recipes as a few may be new to you. These products are the most healthy on this diet, and are available in most natural foods stores or can be purchased online (see the Resources section at the end of this book for website information).

- **Sea salt.** You will notice that we prefer you use Celtic or French sea salts. Traditional table salt usually comes from salt mines, and once mined, it undergoes a refining process that removes the minerals until it is pure sodium chloride. In comparison, Celtic and French sea salts are unrefined so they retain more of the minerals that naturally occur in seawater.
- **Herbamare** is an organic herbal mixture that has been in Europe for decades. It is a blend of herbs, vegetables, and kelp, all organically grown, that are infused fresh (not dried) into sea salt. The herbal mixture can be used to replace salt or to season food. Freeze after opening.
- **Goat cream cheese** has a rich distinct flavor and as close to a perfect food as is possible in nature. The chemical structure of goat's milk is amazingly similar to mother's milk. It is a complete protein containing all the essential amino acids but without the heavy fat content and mucous-producing materials of cow's milk. To learn more about goat milk's special benefits, see the inset opposite.
- **Whey protein powder** is often used as a dietary supplement to improve protein intake. It is a byproduct of the manufacture of cheese and contains all the protein, lactose, vitamins and minerals found in fresh whey. Several cookie recipes call for whey powder. For the best results, we recommend the vanilla bean flavor.

- **Xylitol** is an antimicrobial sugar alternative. It kills yeast, does not promote Candida, and is the best sweetener for a yeast-free diet. Imagine an all-natural sweetener that has one-quarter the carbohydrates and 40 percent less calories than sugar. And instead of being harmful, it fights yeast and has health-giving qualities. What we like most is that xylitol does not cause an insulin response in the body. It does not cause sugar cravings, is teaspoon for teaspoon the same sweetness as sugar, and looks and tastes like sugar. And, it actually helps stabilize blood sugar. This makes it an excellent choice for yeast-free dieters, diabetics, and sugar-intolerant humans (most of us). For more on this healthy, all-natural sugar alternative, read *The Sweet Miracle of Xylitol* (2003).

WHY GOAT'S MILK?

Most of us were brought up on cow's milk and told to drink it every day. Yet goat's milk and the products made from it have special benefits—especially for someone on a yeast-free diet. Here's why we are recommending milk from goats rather than cows.

- **Easier digestibility.** Goat's milk offers superior digestibility to cow's milk. It contains more medium-chain triglycerides (MCTs) than cow's milk. MCTs have a unique ability to provide energy to the human metabolism, as well as to lower, inhibit, and dissolve cholesterol deposits. They actually burn fat. This combination makes it easier for the body's digestive enzymes to break down the milk.
- **Less lactose.** Goat's milk contains approximately 10 percent less lactose (milk sugar) than cow's milk. Lactose like all sugar hosts yeast in the body.
- **Less allergenic.** People with milk intolerance or milk allergy can generally tolerate goat's milk better than cow's milk.
- **Different vitamins and minerals.** Goat's milk is nutritionally superior in some vitamins and minerals to cow's milk. Goat's milk contains more vitamins A, B_3 (niacin), B_6 (pyridoxine), and D than cow's milk, and has a slightly higher content of potassium, copper, and manganese. It is slightly lower in folic acid and vitamin B_{12}, and zinc than that of cow's milk.

HERBAL SEASONINGS AND SAUCES

Here are the herbal seasonings and sauces that will keep you from being bored and fill your foods with great flavor. They can be used in any dish you make. They have been grouped in one section so you can economically buy fresh herbs, mince them, and prepare the combinations—all at the same time. Buy small glass jars, mix the herbs according to the recipes, and freeze them. Then you have them at your fingertips whenever you wish to "spice-up" a meal. The mixtures may be used liberally in recipes.

Why fresh, you may ask. As herbs dry they gather yeast, so for your best health, use fresh or frozen herbs only.

Joan Stott, a patient and friend from North Palm Beach, Florida, contributed the herb mix recipes.

Seasoned Salt

MAKES 25 TEASPOONS • **PHASES 1, 2, 3**

YOU WILL NEED:
3-ounce glass jar with screw-on lid

3 tablespoons French or Celtic sea salt
2 teaspoons fresh thyme, minced
4 teaspoons fresh basil, minced
4 teaspoons fresh tarragon, minced
4 teaspoons fresh rosemary, minced
4 teaspoons fresh flat-leaf parsley, minced

Combine all the ingredients in a glass jar. Shake well each time before using. Freeze the leftover mixture.

Herbes de Provence

MAKES 30 TEASPOONS • **PHASES 1, 2, 3**

YOU WILL NEED:
3-ounce glass jar with screw-on lid

3 tablespoons fresh marjoram, minced
3 tablespoons fresh thyme, minced
3 tablespoons fresh savory, minced
1 teaspoon fresh basil, minced
1 teaspoon fresh rosemary, minced
1/2 teaspoon fresh fennel, minced
1/2 teaspoon fresh sage, minced
1 tablespoon French or Celtic sea salt

Combine all the ingredients in a glass jar. Shake well each time before using. Freeze the leftover mixture.

For poaching fish: Use half the recipe. Wrap all the ingredients in a small cheesecloth bag. Tie the bag and add it to the poaching water.

Herbs for Salad Dressing

MAKES 15 TEASPOONS • **PHASES 1, 2, 3**

YOU WILL NEED:
3-ounce glass jar with screw-on lid

3 tablespoons fresh basil, minced
3 tablespoons fresh flat-leaf parsley, minced
1/2 teaspoon nutmeg, grated
3/4 teaspoon white onion, minced
1/2 teaspoon fresh ginger, finely grated
3 teaspoons French or Celtic sea salt

Combine all the ingredients in a glass jar. Shake well. Freeze the leftover mixture.

Use to season foods or to shake on a salad. For a delicious salad dressing, add the herb mixture to olive oil or an organic oil of your choice, and add lemon juice to taste.

Poultry Rub

MAKES 17 TEASPOONS • **PHASES 1, 2, 3**

YOU WILL NEED:
3-ounce glass jar with screw-on lid

4 teaspoons fresh sage, minced
4 teaspoons fresh thyme, minced
2 teaspoons fresh ginger, minced
2 teaspoons nutmeg, grated
6 teaspoons fresh rosemary, minced
2 teaspoons French or Celtic sea salt
1 teaspoon xylitol

Combine all the ingredients in a glass jar. Shake well each time before using. Freeze the leftover mixture.

Use to flavor poultry recipes, or rub on chicken or turkey before broiling or baking.

Beef Rub

MAKES 14 TEASPOONS • **PHASES 1, 2, 3**

YOU WILL NEED:
3-ounce glass jar with screw-on lid

2 teaspoons fresh garlic, minced
6 teaspoons fresh flat-leaf parsley, minced
2 teaspoons toasted onions, minced
2 teaspoons fresh sage, minced
1/2 teaspoon fresh thyme, minced
2 tablespoons French or Celtic sea salt

Combine all the ingredients in a glass jar. Shake well each time before using. Freeze the leftover mixture.

Use to flavor a recipe, or rub on meats that you broil or bake, just before cooking.

Lemon Barbecue Sauce

MAKES 12 TABLESPOONS • **PHASES 1, 2, 3**

YOU WILL NEED: Small mixing bowl

1 small clove garlic
1/2 teaspoon sea salt
1/2 cup extra virgin olive oil
1/4 cup freshly squeezed lemon juice
2 tablespoons onion, chopped
1/2 teaspoon fresh thyme, minced
1 teaspoon xylitol

Mash the garlic clove in bowl with a fork. Add the salt. Mix in the oil and add the remaining ingredients. Chill to blend the flavors. Excellent on grilled fish.

Clarified Butter (Ghee)

MAKES 1½ CUPS • **PHASES 1, 2, 3**

YOU WILL NEED:
2-cup round-bottom heat-safe container

1 pound unsalted butter

Place the butter into a round-bottom container with outward sloping sides (Pyrex works well; do not use plastic). Melt the butter slowly over low heat. You will observe three layers: a white foamy layer on the top, a white granular layer on the bottom, and a totally clear golden liquid in the middle. This golden liquid is the clarified butter. Once the butter has melted, place the warm container in the refrigerator and allow it to cool and harden.

Remove the hardened butter from the refrigerator and slide it out of the bowl. If necessary, warm the container just enough to loosen the clarified butter. Using a spoon, remove the white foamy top layer and the granular bottom layer. Save the clarified butter center layer for cooking or as a spread.

Lemon Butter

MAKES 5 TABLESPOONS • **PHASES 1, 2, 3**

YOU WILL NEED: Small saucepan

3 tablespoons Clarified Butter (page 66)
1 tablespoon fresh lemon juice
1 tablespoon fresh parsley, minced
½ teaspoon French or Celtic sea salt
Grated peel of half a lemon, washed well before zesting

Melt the butter over low heat. Add the remaining ingredients and blend well.

Garlic Butter/Oil

5 TABLESPOONS • **PHASES 1, 2, 3**

YOU WILL NEED: Small saucepan

1/4 cup Clarified Butter (page 66) or macadamia nut oil

2 cloves of garlic, crushed

1/2 teaspoon fresh chives, minced

French or Celtic sea salt

Melt the butter in a saucepan. Add the garlic and chives. Simmer for 1 minute. Add salt to taste and blend well.

Susan's Yeast-Free Salad Dressing

MAKES 14 TABLESPOONS • **PHASES 1, 2, 3**

YOU WILL NEED:
Blender or food processor

1 cup of hemp oil or flax oil or both combined

2 tablespoon lemon juice

2 to 3 cloves garlic, crushed

1 teaspoon Herbamare

2 teaspoons fresh basil, minced

1/4 teaspoon French or Celtic sea salt or to taste

1 teaspoon dry mustard

Fresh parsley to taste, minced

1 hard-boiled egg, shelled

Place all the ingredients in a blender and blend well. This recipe can be doubled. It will last several days in the refrigerator.

Hollandaise

MAKES 16 TABLESPOONS • **PHASES 1, 2, 3**

YOU WILL NEED:
Double boiler • Whisk or hand mixer

1/2 cup Clarified Butter (page 66)

1/4 teaspoon French or Celtic sea salt

Dash of cayenne pepper

2 tablespoons fresh lemon juice

2/3 cup boiling water

4 egg yolks

Melt the butter in the top of a double boiler over hot (not boiling) water. Stir constantly to keep it creamy. Add the salt, cayenne, lemon juice, and water. Beat constantly with a whisk or hand mixer.

Remove the top from the heat, add egg yolks one at a time and continue to beat until mixture is light and fluffy.

Replace the top on the double boiler over hot water and continue beating until mixture turns glossy and thickens. Cover and keep warm until serving time. (If mixture curdles, beat until smooth.)

Mustard-Dill Sauce

MAKES 4 TABLESPOONS • **PHASES 2, 3**

YOU WILL NEED:
Small mixing bowl • Small whisk

2 tablespoons whipped cream cheese

1 teaspoon powdered mustard

1 tablespoon fresh dill, minced

1 tablespoon Hollandaise (page 68)

1/2 teaspoon xylitol

Blend all ingredients together and refrigerate.

Mayonnaise

MAKES 24 TABLESPOONS • **PHASES 2, 3**

YOU WILL NEED:
Blender or food processor

1 very fresh certified organic egg

1/4 teaspoon dry mustard

1/2 teaspoon French or Celtic sea salt

Pinch white pepper

1/8 teaspoon paprika

1/8 teaspoon xylitol

1 tablespoon fresh lemon juice

1 cup almond oil

Place everything except the oil in a blender and cover. Blend on slow speed. Remove the center plug in cover, and drizzle the oil into the whirling liquid until it is completely emulsified.

BREAKFAST AND BRUNCH

Basic Omelet

SERVES TWO • **PHASES 1, 2, 3**

YOU WILL NEED:
Medium-sized heavy skillet or omelet pan

2 tablespoons Clarified Butter (page 66)

4 large organic eggs

1 tablespoon water

1/2 teaspoon French or Celtic sea salt, or any one of the herb mixes

Melt the butter in a heavy skillet or omelet pan. Tilt the pan to cover with the butter.

Beat the eggs with water and seasoned salt. Pour into the pan and tilt pan to spread the eggs to the edges of pan.

Cook over a low flame until the eggs begin to set. Loosen the eggs from the sides of the pan with a spatula and allow the uncooked egg to flow under the egg pancake.

Tilt the pan again to allow the uncooked eggs to slide to the sides. Carefully fold the outer edges of the omelet into the center to resemble a flat cone. Slide the omelet out of the pan and serve.

You can use any leftover protein or vegetable to fill the omelet before folding it. If you are filling the omelet, spoon the mixture onto the center of the omelet before folding the edges into the center.

Deviled Salmon Eggs

SERVES ONE OR TWO • **PHASES 1, 2, 3**

YOU WILL NEED: Small mixing bowl

3 hard-boiled eggs, shelled

2 ounces fresh poached salmon, flaked

1 teaspoon sesame oil

Juice of 1/2 lemon

1 teaspoon sesame seeds, toasted (optional on Phase 1)

French or Celtic sea salt

Cut the eggs in half lengthwise. Remove the yolks and mash them with the salmon, sesame oil and lemon juice. Sprinkle with the sesame seeds and salt to taste. Spoon the egg mixture into the cavity of egg whites. Cover and use to snack on.

Sweet Fritters

SERVES TWO • **PHASES 1, 2, 3**

YOU WILL NEED:
Electric or hand mixer
Medium-sized baking dish

2 eggs, separated

1 teaspoon xylitol or to taste

3/4 teaspoon cinnamon

2 tablespoons Clarified Butter (page 66)

Preheat the oven to 350°F. Beat the egg whites with the sugar substitute until stiff. Add the cinnamon to the egg yolks, combine well, and fold the yolks into the whites.

Melt the butter in a baking dish. Drop the egg mixture by tablespoonfuls into the hot butter. Bake at 350°F for 20 minutes.

Tasty Egg Pancakes with Grass-Fed Beef

SERVES TWO • **PHASES 1, 2, 3**

YOU WILL NEED: Small heavy skillet

½ pound grass-fed beef, ground
3 egg yolks, lightly beaten
1 teaspoon lemon juice
⅛ small onion, grated
1 teaspoon Beef Rub (page 65)
¼ teaspoon dry mustard
French or Celtic sea salt to taste
3 egg whites, beaten stiff
2 tablespoons macadamia nut oil

Mix the first seven ingredients together in a glass bowl. Fold in the egg whites. Blend well.

Warm the oil in a skillet, covering the bottom of it with the oil. Drop the mixture on the skillet by tablespoonfuls. Brown on one side, turn and brown on the other side.

Ginger Lemonade

A great way to start your day

MAKES 4 TO 6 CUPS • **PHASES 1, 2, 3**

YOU WILL NEED:
Reamer or juicer • Pitcher

2 pieces of fresh ginger root (about ¼ cup), peeled and grated
Freshly squeezed juice of 3 large lemons
4 cups water
Xylitol and water to taste

Peel and slice the ginger. Place it in a pot with 4 cups water. Bring the mixture to a boil and simmer covered for at least an hour.

Add water and xylitol to taste. This may be very strong for you. Adding water and sweetening it will make it your perfect, healthy, go-to drink. Cool the drink to room temperature. Squeeze in the juice of three lemons. Pour into a pitcher and refrigerate. The lemonade may be consumed hot or cold.

Popovers

Not for the first time cook, but worth the effort

MAKES SIX • **PHASES 2, 3**

YOU WILL NEED:
Popover pan with 6 sections or heavy muffin pan

1/2 cup whey protein

2 tablespoon Clarified Butter (page 66), melted

1 1/2 cups goat's milk

2 eggs

1/4 teaspoon French or Celtic sea salt

6 teaspoons coconut oil

Preheat the oven to 425°F. Grease the popover cups. Heat in preheated oven for 10 minutes.

Whisk together whey protein, melted butter, goat's milk, eggs, and sea salt.

Place one teaspoon of coconut oil in each cup. Immediately, pour the batter evenly into the hot cups until two-thirds full.

Bake a 450°F for 15 minutes. Reduce the heat to 325°F, and continue baking for another 12 minutes. Serve simply with Clarified Butter, or remove the top and fill with your favorite salad or meat.

For variety, add 1 tablespoon of fresh parsley or dill to the batter before cooking. This is the best bread substitute I know. Simply delicious.

Sausage Frittata

SERVES FOUR • **PHASE 3**

YOU WILL NEED:
9- x 9-inch casserole dish
Large skillet

2 links organic Italian turkey sausage
2 cloves garlic, minced
3 shallots, chopped
2 scallions, sliced
1/2 red pepper, diced (optional)
10 grape tomatoes, cut in quarters
1/4 cup zucchini, shredded
2 tablespoons parsley, chopped
1 teaspoon Herbamare
Pinch French or Celtic sea salt and white pepper
Several drops hot pepper sauce (optional)
6 eggs, well beaten

Preheat the oven to 350°F. Squeeze the sausage out of the casing into the skillet. Break it up into small pieces as it cooks. When the sausage is almost browned on all sides, add the garlic, shallots, and red pepper. Cook until well browned.

Remove the mixture from the skillet to a buttered casserole dish. Mix in the grape tomatoes and shredded zucchini, parsley, and Herbamare.

Beat the salt, pepper, and hot pepper (if using) sauce into eggs, and pour the eggs over the sausage mixture.

Bake at 350°F for 35 to 40 minutes until firm.

Fresh Raspberry Omelet

SERVES FOUR • **PHASE 3**

YOU WILL NEED:
1 small bowl • 1 medium-sized bowl
Medium-sized non-stick omelet pan with cover

3 tablespoons fresh tarragon, minced, or 2 tablespoons dried from freezer

3 ounces goat cream cheese, room temperature

8 eggs

3 tablespoons spring water

1 teaspoon Seasoned Salt (page 62) or Herbamare

2 tablespoons butter

6 ounces fresh raspberries

2 ounces sliced almonds, lightly toasted

1 grapefruit, sectioned, for garnish (optional)

In a small bowl, sprinkle the tarragon over the cream cheese. Blend well with a fork. Form the cream cheese mixture into small balls and set aside.

Break the eggs into a medium-sized bowl. Add the water and seasoned salt. Beat well.

Melt the butter in an omelet pan over medium heat. Pour the egg mixture into the pan, and tilt the pan to cover the bottom with the eggs. Evenly distribute the cream cheese balls, raspberries, and almonds (reserve 2 tablespoons for garnish) over the surface of the eggs. Reduce the heat to medium-low and cover the pan. Cook for 3 to 5 minutes or to the way you like your eggs cooked. Fold the egg mixture in half using a rubber spatula. Place the omelet on a plate and garnish with the remaining almonds, and fan out four grapefruit slices on one side of the omelet. This omelet is beautiful to look at, and a special taste treat.

Ginger, Pumpkin Seed, and Swiss-Surprise Omelet

SERVES ONE (double the recipe for two) • **PHASE 3**

YOU WILL NEED:
Non-stick omelet pan
Rubber spatula

1 tablespoon coconut butter

1 tablespoon fresh ginger, peeled and chopped

1 tablespoon unsalted pumpkin seeds

4 sugar snap peas, deveined and quartered

2 large eggs

2 tablespoons Swiss cheese, grated

Seasoned Salt to taste (page 62)

Melt the coconut butter in an omelet pan over medium heat. Add the ginger, pumpkin seeds, and peas. Sauté until the ginger becomes soft (about two minutes.)

Beat the eggs with the cheese and salt. Add the egg mixture to an omelet pan, and shake the pan to distribute the ginger mixture evenly. Allow the omelet to set, lifting edges with a rubber spatula to permit the uncooked egg to flow to the bottom of the pan. Cook until set, but not dry. Fold the omelet in half, and slide onto a plate.

STOCKS

Fish Stock

4 CUPS • **PHASES 1, 2, 3**

YOU WILL NEED:
2-quart saucepan or stockpot
Storage containers

2 tablespoons sesame oil

2 tablespoons Clarified Butter (page 66)

1 large onion, sliced

1 small turnip, peeled and diced

2 stalks celery, chopped

3 pounds fresh flounder or halibut or other fish, fish bones, or fish heads (shrimp and lobster shells can be substituted)

1 teaspoon fresh lemon juice

4 sprigs fresh parsley

4 whole peppercorns

Cold water to cover

1 tablespoon Herbamare

French or Celtic sea salt to taste

Heat the butter and oil in a heavy-bottomed 2-quart saucepan or pot. Add the onion and sauté over medium heat until tender. Add the turnip and celery, and sauté until golden brown. Add the fish, lemon juice, parsley, and peppercorns and cover with 2 inches of cold water.

Slowly bring the stock to a simmer, skimming the top of fat when necessary. Simmer gently for 30 minutes. Remove from the heat. Correct the seasonings with Herbamare and salt to taste. Strain and refrigerate. This stock may be frozen.

Rich Beef Stock

MAKES APPROXIMATELY 4 CUPS • **PHASES 1, 2, 3**

YOU WILL NEED:

A saucepan or stockpot precisely the size of the ingredients you are putting into it

Ice trays

6 pounds beef oxtail

1 large yellow onion, chopped

1 green pepper, cored and quartered

2 tablespoons Herbes de Provence (page 63)

Water just to cover

Place the beef tails side by side in saucepan or stockpot. Top with the onion, pepper, and herb mixture. Add just enough water to cover the ingredients. Simmer for 3 to 4 hours (until the beef pulls easily from the bone). Cool. Remove the vegetables and discard. Refrigerate overnight.

The next day skim the fat from the top. Remove the tail from the beef gel and discard (it usually is stringy and not flavorful).

Push the remaining gel through a strainer, place it in ice trays, and freeze. You will use this in many dishes in this book—one rich beef stock cube at a time.

Rich Chicken Stock

MAKES APPROXIMATELY 6 CUPS • **PHASES 1, 2, 3**

YOU WILL NEED:
A saucepan or stockpot precisely the size of the ingredients you are putting into it
Ice trays

3 pounds organic or free-range chicken, quartered (add neck and organs to pot)

6 whole green onions

1 turnip, peeled and quartered

Enough spring water to fill saucepan

French or Celtic sea salt, to taste

White pepper to taste

Arrange the chicken to fill the saucepan or stockpot. Chop the tops of the green onions and add to the pan. Lay the bottom half of the green onions on top of the chicken Add the turnips and water. Bring to a slow boil. Turn the heat down to low, and simmer for two hours (until the chicken pulls easily from the bone). Cool. Refrigerate intact overnight.

The next day skim the fat from the top. Remove the chicken. Skin the chicken and remove from the bone to snack on.

Push the remaining stock through a strainer, place it in ice trays and freeze. You will use this in many dishes in this book—one rich chicken stock cube at a time.

Vegetable Rich Stock

This can be eaten as a soup

MAKES APPROXIMATELY TEN 1-CUP SERVINGS • **PHASES 1, 2, 3**

YOU WILL NEED: Large stockpot
Blender or food processor • Storage containers

1/3 cup macadamia nut oil
2 large onions, chopped
1 small leek, sliced
2 tablespoons garlic, chopped
1 medium zucchini, chopped
1 medium yellow squash, chopped
1/2 cup fresh fennel, chopped
1/3 cup fresh turnip, peeled and chopped
1 cup fresh spinach, chopped
3 stalks celery, chopped
1 cup tomatoes, chopped
1 cup fresh flat-leaf parsley, chopped
1 teaspoon fresh oregano
1 teaspoon fresh rosemary
1 teaspoon fresh sage
1 teaspoon fresh tarragon
1 teaspoon fresh thyme
1/2 teaspoon nutmeg, freshly grated
1 tablespoon French or Celtic sea salt
6 cups water

Heat the oil in a stockpot. Add the onions, leek, and garlic. Sauté the mixture over medium heat for several minutes until browned. Stir in the zucchini, yellow squash, fennel, turnip, spinach, celery, tomatoes, fresh herbs, nutmeg, salt, and pepper. Add water.

Bring to a boil, and then turn heat down to simmer. Cover. Simmer for 1 hour, stirring occasionally.

Remove from heat and allow to cool.

Puree in a blender 2 cups at a time. Place in 1-cup containers and ice trays and freeze.

APPETIZERS AND SNACKS

Finger-Lickin' Good Roasted Garlic

SERVES TWO • **PHASES 1, 2, 3**

YOU WILL NEED: Small baking dish

1 head elephant garlic or 1 large head garlic, unpeeled

1 tablespoon extra virgin olive oil

Preheat the oven 350°F. Rub the garlic bulb with oil and place it in a baking dish. Bake for 30 minutes. Cool. Squeeze the soft garlic out of the skin to eat.

Crabby, Crabby, Crabby Crab Cakes

The ultimate crab cake

MAKES SIXTEEN APPETIZERS OR FOUR DINNER-SIZED CRAB CAKES
PHASES 2, 3

YOU WILL NEED: Food processor
Medium-sized mixing bowl • Medium-sized skillet

1/2 pound lump crabmeat*

3/4 cup pecans, finely ground

1 tablespoon minced fresh chives or one teaspoon dried

2 tablespoons goat cream cheese

Herbamare

3 heaping tablespoons coconut butter

6 large shallots, sliced

16 leaves flat-leaf parsley

Place the crabmeat in a mixing bowl. Add half the crushed pecans, Herbamare to taste, chives, and cream cheese. Blend well.

Heat the coconut butter in a skillet. Add the shallots. Sauté over medium heat until soft and lightly colored.

Roll the crabmeat mixture into balls the size of walnuts. Roll the crab balls in the remaining crushed pecans. Flatten the balls into the shape of small burgers, and place them in the coconut butter. Cover and cook for 4 minutes. Remove the cover, gently turn each crab cake over (you don't want it to fall apart) and allow it to brown on the other side for one minute. Carefully remove the crab cakes from the pan, and spoon the pan juices over them. Allow the cakes to sit for 5 minutes before serving. Garnish the appetizers with a piece of flat-leaf parsley.

To serve as a main dish, use 1/2 cup pecans and 2 tablespoons coconut butter. Divide the crab mixture into four burger-shaped crab cakes. When all the crab cakes have been placed in the coconut butter, cover the pan and allow the crab to cook through for 5 minutes. Turn once and cook for 3 minutes on the other side. Carefully remove from pan, and spoon the pan juices over them. Allow the cakes to sit for 5 minutes before serving. Garnish with parsley leaves.

*Note: Crab substitute will not give you the flaky texture or flavor of this delicious dish made with real lump crabmeat. If for some reason you cannot use real crabmeat, use white albacore tuna that has been packed in water.

Spicy, Spicy, Spicy Crab Cakes

MAKES SIXTEEN APPETIZERS OR FOUR DINNER-SIZED CRAB CAKES

PHASES 2, 3

YOU WILL NEED: Blender or food processor
Medium-sized mixing bowl • Medium-sized skillet

1/2 pound lump crabmeat*

2 tablespoons macadamia nut butter

1/3 red pepper, diced

¼ cup green onions, minced

⅛ teaspoon cayenne pepper or red pepper, ground

Seasoned Salt (page 62)

½ cup macadamia nuts, finely ground

3 heaping tablespoons coconut butter

Place the crabmeat in a mixing bowl. Add the macadamia nut butter, red pepper, green onions, cayenne, and seasoned salt to taste. Blend well.

Put the nuts in a food processor and grind until finely ground.

Melt the coconut butter in a skillet over medium heat.

Roll the crabmeat mixture into 16 balls, the size of walnuts. Roll the crab balls in the crushed macadamia nuts. Flatten the balls into the shape of small burgers, and place in the coconut butter. When all the crab cakes have been placed in the coconut butter, cover the pan and allow to cook through for 3 minutes. Remove the cover, gently turn each crab cake over (you don't want it to fall apart) and allow it to brown on the other side for 1 minute. Carefully remove from pan, and spoon pan juices over the crab cakes. Allow them to cool for 5 minutes before serving.

To serve as a main dish, divide the crab mixture into four burger-shaped crab cakes. When all the crab cakes have been placed in the coconut butter, cover the pan and allow to cook through for 5 minutes. Remove the cover, gently turn each crab cake over (you don't want it to fall apart) and allow it to brown on the other side for 3 minutes. Carefully remove from pan, and spoon pan juices over the crab cakes. Allow them to cool for 5 minutes before serving.

*Note: Crab substitute will not give you the flaky texture or flavor of this delicious dish made with real lump crabmeat. If for some reason you cannot use real crabmeat, use white albacore tuna that has been packed in water.

Garlic Walnuts

MAKES 1/2 CUP • **PHASES 2, 3**

YOU WILL NEED: Small skillet

2 tablespoons Garlic Butter/Oil (page 67)

1/2 cup walnuts halves

1 tablespoon garlic, minced

Heat the oil in a skillet over medium heat. Add the walnuts and toss until coated well with the oil. Sprinkle garlic over the walnuts. Toss again. Remove from the skillet and cool on a paper towel.

Always refrigerate nuts. They can easily become rancid at room temperature.

Sweet Pecans

MAKES 1/2 CUP • **PHASES 2, 3**

YOU WILL NEED: Small skillet

2 tablespoons butter

1/2 cup pecan halves

1 tablespoon xylitol

Melt the butter in a skillet. Add the pecans and toss until coated well with butter. Sprinkle xylitol over the pecans. Toss again. Remove from the skillet and cool on a paper towel.

Always refrigerate nuts. They can easily become rancid at room temperature.

So You Think You Can't Eat Pizza

When only pizza will do, try this

SERVES FOUR • **PHASES 2, 3**

YOU WILL NEED: Small bowl
12-inch pizza pan or springform pan

Crust

1/2 cup unflavored whey protein powder
1 egg
2 tablespoons extra virgin olive oil
5 tablespoons goat's milk
1/8 teaspoon French or Celtic sea salt
1/2 teaspoon fresh or frozen oregano, minced
1/2 teaspoon non-aluminum baking powder

Topping

3/4 to 1 cup tomato sauce
2 cups goat cheese, shredded
1 cup of your favorite vegetables, chopped in no larger than 1-inch pieces
1 teaspoon fresh oregano, minced
1/2 teaspoon fresh garlic, minced

Preheat the oven to 350°F. Put the crust ingredients into a bowl and whisk until the mixture forms a thin batter.

Generously oil a 12-inch pizza pan. Pour in the batter and tilt to cover the bottom. Place the pan on the middle rack of an oven, and bake for 10 minutes.

Carefully remove the crust from the pan and turn over in the pan, so the browned side is facing up. Spread the sauce over the surface of the crust, being careful to cover the edges. Distribute one cup of the cheese evenly. Add the vegetables. Top with second cup of cheese. Sprinkle on the oregano and garlic.

Place on top rack of oven, and bake for 15 minutes or until the cheese begins to brown.

Spicy Almonds

MAKES 1/2 CUP • **PHASES 2, 3**

YOU WILL NEED: Small skillet

2 tablespoons extra virgin olive oil

1/2 cup almonds

1 tablespoon of your favorite Herbal Mixture or Rub (pages 62–65)

Heat the oil in a skillet. Add the almonds and toss until coated well with oil. Sprinkle the herb mixture or rub over the almonds. Toss again. Remove from the skillet and cool on a paper towel.

Always refrigerate all nuts. They can easily become rancid at room temperature.

Parmesan Crackers

When you need to taste crunch

MAKES 40 CRACKERS • **PHASE 3**

YOU WILL NEED: Mixing bowl • Cookie sheet
Parchment paper • Cooling rack

1 cup whey protein powder

1 teaspoon baking powder

1/2 teaspoon sea salt

1 egg

1/4 cup water

1/2 cup grated Parmesan cheese

2 tablespoons Clarified Butter (page 66)

Preheat the oven to 325°F. Mix the whey powder, baking powder, salt, egg, water, and grated cheese together in a mixing bowl.

Place the parchment paper on a cookie sheet, and grease it with the melted butter.

Drop the batter by teaspoonfuls onto the paper, keeping them 3 inches apart.

Bake 10 to 12 minutes, until golden, rotating the pan 180° degrees halfway through the cooking time. Remove to a cooling rack.

Coconut Shrimp with Peach Sauce

MAKES 1 DOZEN • **PHASE 3**

YOU WILL NEED: ***Large, deep skillet***
3 small bowls • Paper bag
Blender or food processor

Shrimp

Coconut oil

12 jumbo shrimp, shelled and deveined

2 eggs, beaten

1 cup shredded coconut

Melt enough coconut oil in a skillet to measure 2 inches deep. Dip the shrimp into egg, then roll in enough shredded coconut to coat the shrimp. Deep fry the shrimp in the oil until golden brown (about 2 minutes if the oil is very hot). Remove the shrimp from the oil with a slotted spoon. Drain on paper bag. Serve covered with Peach Sauce (see below).

Peach Sauce

3 medium-ripe peaches, peeled and pitted

1/4 teaspoon lemon juice

1/2 teaspoon xylitol

Place all the ingredients in a blender. Blend until smooth.

SOUPS

The Levin's Chicken Soup

SERVES FOUR • **PHASES 1, 2, 3**

YOU WILL NEED: Large stockpot

1 organic chicken, cut into eight pieces
Poultry Rub (page 64)
Water to cover chicken
3 to 4 cloves garlic, minced
2 sprigs fresh dill
French or Celtic sea salt
6 stalks of celery, diced
2 onions, quartered
2 fresh turnips, peeled and quartered

Season the chicken with the Poultry Rub. Place it in the stockpot. Cover the chicken with water. Add the garlic, dill, and salt to taste. Next add the vegetables. Bring to a boil, then lower to a simmer. Cook for about 2 hours. Remove from the heat and allow to cool.

Remove the vegetables from the liquid with a slotted spoon. Throw away the dill, and puree the vegetables in a food processor or blender, or keep as they were sliced. Serve warm.

Garlic Soup

Add any protein you wish

SERVES FOUR • **PHASES 1, 2, 3**

YOU WILL NEED: Large stockpot

6 large cloves garlic, minced

1/4 cup extra virgin olive oil

4 egg yolks

2 quarts Vegetable Stock (page 80) or store-bought, organic, sugar-free vegetable broth, simmering

2 teaspoons French or Celtic sea salt

1 tablespoon Herbes de Provence (page 63)

1 cup any animal protein, cooked and diced

Add the garlic, oil, and egg yolks to the simmering stock. Add the salt, herbs, and protein. Simmer for 1/2 hour.

Soup Noodles

These can be added to any soup

SERVES TWO • **PHASES 1, 2, 3**

YOU WILL NEED: Cookie sheet with sides

3 tablespoons Clarified Butter (page 66)

2 eggs, room temperature and separated

1/4 teaspoon Seasoned Salt (page 62)

Preheat the oven to 350°F. Melt the butter on a cookie sheet.

Beat the egg whites with the salt until stiff. Beat the yolks with a fork. Carefully fold the whites into the yolks; try not to break down the whites.

Spread the mixture on the cookie sheet. Bake for 10 minutes or until light brown. Cool on a rack. Slice into "noodles" and use in soups.

Gently Flavored Cauliflower Soup

SERVES SIX • **PHASES 2, 3**

YOU WILL NEED:
3-quart saucepan or stockpot
Blender or food processor

1 head of cauliflower, trimmed and diced

$1^1/_2$ tablespoons coriander

$^1/_2$ tablespoon nutmeg

1 organic lemon, juice and grated rind

1 cup goat's milk

2 cups Rich Vegetable Stock (page 80) or store-bought, organic, sugar-free vegetable stock

1 cup flat-leaf parsley, chopped

1 cup walnuts, coarsely chopped

$1^1/_2$ tablespoons Herbamare, or to taste

Boil the cauliflower pieces in 2 inches of water until tender (about 10 minutes.) Reserve the cooking water. Set aside 1 cup of the cooked cauliflower pieces.

Puree the rest of the cooked cauliflower, reserved cooking water, coriander, nutmeg, and lemon juice in a blender. Return the puree to the saucepan or stockpot, add the milk, vegetable stock, parsley, remaining cup of cooked cauliflower, walnuts, lemon zest, and Herbamare. Heat to a simmer. Do not boil. Ladle into six soup bowls. Serve hot. Leftovers may be served hot or cold.

Salmon Chowder

A meal in a bowl

SERVES FOUR • **PHASES 2, 3**

YOU WILL NEED:
Large non-stick skillet with cover

Grill

2 teaspoons coconut butter

1 large leek top, chopped

1/4 green pepper, chopped (optional)

3 cloves garlic, minced

1 parsnip, diced

2 cups Rich Chicken Stock (page 79) or store-bought, organic, sugar-free chicken broth

1 medium-sized zucchini, peeled and diced

1 teaspoon fresh dill, chopped

1/2 teaspoon curry

1 teaspoon Herbamare

1/2 cup almond milk

1 pound fresh salmon filet, sprinkled with lemon juice

1/4 cup pine nuts, toasted

Melt the coconut butter over medium heat in the bottom of a skillet. Add the leek, green pepper, garlic, and parsnip. Sauté for 5 minutes. Add the broth, zucchini, and dill. Sprinkle with curry powder and Herbamare. Cover and allow to simmer for 20 minutes.

While the chowder is cooking, grill the salmon, using either an indoor or outdoor grill, or a non-stick grill pan.

When the vegetables are tender (not mushy), remove the pan from the heat and whisk in the almond milk. Ladle the vegetable mixture into four large soup bowls. Divide the salmon into four equal pieces and flake it over the top of each bowl. Garnish with the toasted pine nuts.

Split Pea Soup

SERVES FOUR • **PHASES 2, 3**

YOU WILL NEED:
Medium-sized heavy skillet or stockpot

1 cup onion, chopped

1 teaspoon macadamia nut oil

1 pound dried split peas, washed well

1 pound ham bone

Water to cover

1/4 teaspoon French or Celtic sea salt

2 teaspoons Herbes de Provence (page 63)

Heat the oil in a medium-sized skillet or stockpot over medium heat. Sauté the onions until soft and lightly colored. Add the split peas, ham bone, and enough water to cover ingredients; season with the salt and herbs.

Cover and cook for about 2 hours or until there are no whole peas left and the mixture is a green liquid. Set aside to cool. While the soup is cooking, check to see if water has evaporated. You may need to add more water as it continues to cook. Once the soup has thickened, warm and serve.

VEGETABLES

Oven-Roasted Vegetables

SERVES FOUR • **PHASES 1, 2, 3**

YOU WILL NEED:
Baking sheet • Parchment paper

2 baby eggplant, sliced lengthwise into 1/8-inch slices

1 zucchini, sliced into 1/8-inch slices

4 cloves of garlic or more to taste

1 large green pepper, sliced into 1/8-inch slices

1 large red pepper, sliced into 1/8-inch slices

2 tablespoons macadamia nut oil

1 teaspoon fresh or frozen thyme, minced

1 teaspoon fresh or frozen oregano, minced

Preheat the oven to 400°F. Place the vegetables on a baking sheet lined with parchment paper and toss together with the oil and herbs. Roast for 1/2 hour until tender, stirring occasionally. Make certain not to burn. The vegetables may be served with Lemon Barbecue Sauce (page 65).

Leftovers can be wrapped and saved in refrigerator. They make a great lunch and are good cold or warm.

Latkas

A taste surprise—try these and freeze leftovers—
they will be a favorite

SERVES FOUR • **PHASES 1, 2, 3**

YOU WILL NEED: Medium-sized mixing bowl
Large skillet • Paper bag

4 cups celery root, peeled and grated

2 eggs, lightly beaten

1 medium onion, thinly sliced

1 heaping teaspoon Herbamare

1/4 cup coconut butter

Beat the celery root, eggs, onion, and Herbamare together in a medium-sized bowl.

Melt the coconut oil in the skillet. Heat until very hot. Carefully drop the celery root mixture by tablespoons into the hot oil. Allow each latka to brown on one side for 2 minutes, turn with a slotted spatula, and brown on the other side for another 2 minutes. Remove to a paper bag to drain and crisp.

Spaghetti the Squash Way

SERVES EIGHT • **PHASES 1, 2, 3**

YOU WILL NEED: Roasting pan

1 large spaghetti squash

Preheat the oven to 350°F. Using a sharp knife, make 20 straight cuts into squash. Place it in a roasting pan and bake for 1 1/2 hours. Remove from the oven and cool.

Cut the squash in half, remove the seeds, and pull out the "spaghetti." Serve with Lemon Barbecue Sauce (page 65).

Asparagus Gone Nuts

SERVES FOUR • **PHASES 2, 3**

YOU WILL NEED:
Large skillet

1 bunch asparagus, trimmed
2 tablespoons coconut butter
4 large cloves garlic, minced
1/2 cup fresh basil, chopped
1/4 cup walnuts, chopped
4-ounce log goat cheese
2 teaspoons Herbamare

Wash and trim the asparagus. Heat the coconut oil over medium heat in a skillet. Tilt the pan until the bottom is covered with melted coconut butter. Place the asparagus in the pan and sear on all sides. Remove the asparagus from the pan and set aside.

Add the garlic, basil, and walnuts to pan. Sauté them until the garlic turns golden brown.

Return the asparagus to the pan, top with the goat cheese and allow it to warm. Sprinkle with Herbamare. Cover the skillet, and keep asparagus warm until ready to serve.

Crunchy Bok Choy

SERVES FOUR • **PHASES 2, 3**

YOU WILL NEED: Medium-sized skillet

6 tablespoons sesame oil

1 cup red onion, diced

1 cup pecans, chopped

4 small bok choy (Chinese cabbage), sliced in half lengthwise

Sauté the onion and pecans in 3 tablespoons of the sesame oil until the onions become transparent. Remove the onions and nuts from the pan and cover to keep them warm. Add the remaining sesame oil to the pan and add the bok choy. Sauté until tender.

Place on a serving dish, and top with the onion-nut mixture.

Zucchini in Sweet Peanut Sauce

SERVES FOUR • **PHASES 2, 3**

YOU WILL NEED: Food processor
Medium-sized skillet

$^{1}/_{4}$ cup macadamia nut oil

4 cloves garlic, minced

$^{1}/_{2}$ cup peanuts, finely chopped

1 tablespoon xylitol

1 pound zucchini, cut into $^{1}/_{8}$-inch slices

Put the nuts in a food processor and finely ground. Heat the nut oil in a skillet over medium-high heat. Sauté the garlic in the oil until it begins to brown. Add the peanuts and sprinkle with xylitol. Sauté until the peanuts absorb the oil. Add the zucchini and toss until it is well coated and tender. Serve immediately.

Caponata

A healthy, tasty veggie snack or side dish

MAKES 2 CUPS • **PHASE 3**

YOU WILL NEED: ***Medium-sized skillet***

1/4 cup extra virgin olive oil

1 1/4 pounds eggplant, diced

1 medium onion, diced

2 celery stalks, diced

12 pitted green olives, diced

4 plum tomatoes, diced

1/4 cup lemon juice

1 tablespoon xylitol

1/4 cup pine nuts, lightly toasted

2 tablespoons tomato paste

1/4 cup flat-leaf parsley, chopped

2 teaspoons fresh oregano, minced

Herbamare

Dice the vegetables. Place 2 tablespoons of the olive oil in a heavy skillet. Warm over a medium heat and add the diced eggplant. Sauté the eggplant about 5 minutes until it is soft and cooked through. Remove to a bowl.

Return the skillet to the heat. Add 2 tablespoons more of olive oil and the diced onions and celery. Cook for 5 minutes, stirring occasionally.

Add the olives, tomatoes, lemon juice, xylitol, and pine nuts. Mix well and add the tomato paste. Stir to combine. Add the parsley and oregano. Stir again. Cover and allow to simmer for 10 minutes. Cool to room temperature and refrigerate at least over night.

When ready to serve, season with Herbamare to taste. This dish will keep in the refrigerator for a week or more and can be frozen.

SALADS

Green Bean Salad

SERVES SIX • **PHASES 1, 2, 3**

YOU WILL NEED: Saucepan
Small mixing bowl • Storage container

1 pound fresh green beans
1/2 cup water
1/3 cup lemon juice
1/2 cup extra virgin olive oil
1/2 teaspoon French or Celtic sea salt
3 tablespoons onion, thinly sliced
2 cloves garlic, minced
1/2 teaspoon fresh oregano, minced
1 teaspoon fresh flat-leaf parsley, minced

Wash the beans, and break off and discard the ends. Place the beans in a saucepan with the water. Simmer for 10 minutes. Reserve 1/3 cup water and discard the rest.

Combine the reserved water, lemon juice, sea salt, onion, oregano, and parsley in a bowl. Whisk in the olive oil. Pour the dressing over the beans. Store in a covered container and chill overnight. Remove the beans from the marinade when ready to serve.

4 x 3 Salad

You create it!

SERVES EIGHT BUT MAY BE MADE FOR ONE OR A CROWD

PHASE 2 (WITHOUT FRUIT), PHASE 3 (WITH FRUIT)

YOU WILL NEED: Small non-stick skillet
Large salad bowl

3 cups of your three favorite lettuces (1 cup each), washed and dry

1 1/2 cups of your three favorite veggies (1/2 cup each), diced

3/4 cup of your three favorite low-carbohydrate fruits (1/4 cup each), diced

6 tablespoons of your three favorite nuts or seeds (2 tablespoons each), toasted

1 tablespoon Garlic Butter/Oil (page 67)

2 cups Susan's Yeast-Free Salad Dressing (optional, page 67)

Rip the dry lettuce into bite-sized pieces and place in a salad bowl. Toss in veggies (except the tomatoes if using) and the fruit. At this point the salad can be refrigerated.

When ready to serve, warm the garlic oil in a small non-stick skillet. Add the nuts or seeds and sauté for 3 minutes. Toss into salad. Add tomatoes if using them.

This salad almost doesn't need a dressing. If you want to dress it, use 1/4 cup per person of Susan's Yeast-Free Salad Dressing.

Favorite Chicken Salad

SERVES SIX • **PHASES 2, 3**

YOU WILL NEED: Medium mixing bowl

Meat from 1/2 leftover chicken, chunked
(preferably chicken leftover from Rich Chicken Stock on page 79)

2 tablespoons Mayonnaise (page 69)

1/2 cup walnuts, chopped

1 medium stalk celery, minced

1 tablespoon fresh tarragon, minced

1 tablespoon of your favorite herb mixture or Herbamare

Place the chicken in a bowl. Spoon the mayonnaise on top. Add the nuts, celery, and herbs to center of mayo. Blend well and then toss with the chicken until the meat is well coated. Refrigerate for one hour before serving.

Vermont Salad

SERVES FOUR • **PHASES 2, 3**

YOU WILL NEED: Salad bowl
Small mixing bowl

Salad

8 cups mesclun greens, washed and dried

2 endives, cut in eights

3 large daikon radishes, cut in 1/2-inch cubes

1/2 cup walnuts, coarsely chopped

2 ounces goat cheese, crumbled

1/2 cup red onion, thinly sliced

1/2 cup edamame beans, steamed until soft

Dressing

Juice of 1 lemon

1/2 cup walnut oil

2 teaspoons maple extract

1/4 cup xylitol

Sea salt and pepper

Toss the mesclun, endive, daikon, walnuts, goat cheese, onion, and edamame together in the salad bowl.

Whisk together the lemon juice, oil, maple extract, and xylitol in a bowl. Salt and pepper to taste. Pour dressing over the salad just before serving, and toss.

Thousand Island Dressing

MAKES 1 CUP OR FOUR 1/4-CUP SERVINGS • **PHASES 2, 3**

YOU WILL NEED:
Food processor • Storage jar

3/4 cup Mayonnaise (page 69)

1 scallion, white part plus some of the firm green, chopped

1 plum tomato, seeded, juiced, and quartered

1 teaspoon fresh garlic, minced

2 tablespoons extra virgin olive oil

1 tablespoon lemon juice

3 tablespoons cucumber, finely diced

Sea salt or Herbamare

Place the mayonnaise, scallion, tomato, garlic, olive oil, and lemon juice in the food processor, and pulse until the vegetables are finely chopped. Add the cucumber and chop on low speed until just to mix. Add salt or Herbamare to taste.

MAIN DISHES: RED MEAT AND ROASTS

Veal Roast

SERVES SIX • **PHASES 1, 2, 3**

YOU WILL NEED:
Covered roasting pan large enough to fit the meats

4 to 5 pounds veal roast (breast is my favorite cut)

2 tablespoons Beef Rub (page 65)

2 cloves garlic, sliced into 8 pieces

3 tablespoons organic red palm oil

4 tablespoons onion, chopped

2 celery stalks, diced

1/2 cup of any other permitted vegetable, diced

1/2 cup Rich Chicken Stock (page 79) or store-bought, organic, sugar-free chicken broth

Preheat the oven to 325°F. Rub the Beef Rub onto the veal. Cut eight incisions in the veal and stuff the garlic into the incisions.

Heat the oil in a roasting pan and brown the veal on all sides. Add the onions, celery, (other vegetables), and broth. Cover the pan and cook in the oven for 30 minutes per pound. Open the oven to baste every half hour.

When cooked, remove the roast from the pan and allow it to set for 10 minutes before carving. Remove the vegetables from the pan juices, skim off the fat, and pour the pan juices over the sliced veal.

Savory Leg of Lamb

SERVES SIX • **PHASES 1, 2, 3**

YOU WILL NEED:
Wooden chopping bowl and chopper
Large skillet • Roasting pan

2 teaspoons fresh thyme, minced, or 2 teaspoons dried

4 cloves garlic, minced

2 teaspoons fresh rosemary, minced

1 tablespoon fresh oregano, minced, or 1 teaspoon dried

3 pounds boneless leg of lamb

3 tablespoons extra virgin olive oil

1 tablespoon lemon juice

White pepper (optional)

Preheat the oven to 350°F. Place the thyme, garlic, rosemary, and oregano in a chopping bowl and chop until well blended. Add 1 teaspoon of the olive oil and blend well. Set aside.

Heat the remaining oil in a skillet. Add the lemon juice and pepper if using. Simmer the mixture for 5 minutes. Turn up the heat and place the lamb in the liquid. Turn the lamb until it absorbs most of the marinade. Remove the lamb from pan.

Rub the lamb with the herb mixture and place it in a roasting pan. Cover with the remaining marinade, and roast in an oven for 15 minutes per pound (allow about 1 hour for a 3-pound medium-rare roast). Baste every 20 minutes. Remove from the oven and keep warm. Allow the lamb to set for 15 minutes before serving.

Brisket of Beef

Make this in advance and use it to snack on

SERVES SIX TO EIGHT • **PHASES 1, 2, 3**

YOU WILL NEED:
Dutch oven or stainless steel crockpot
Parchment paper

4 to 5 pounds fresh-cut brisket, first cut (organic or Kosher)

4 large cloves garlic, crushed

Beef Rub (page 65)

3 onions, diced

2 tablespoons macadamia nut oil

French or Celtic sea salt

7 celery stalks, diced

1 red pepper, diced

1 green pepper, diced

2 cups Rich Beef Stock (page 78) or store-bought, organic, sugar-free beef broth

Preheat the oven to 375°F. Remove any excess fat from the brisket. Season the brisket by rubbing it with the Beef Rub and garlic to taste. Wrap it in parchment paper and refrigerate it over night (seasoned meat can keep in the refrigerator for up to three days). When you are ready to cook the brisket, bring it to room temperature.

Place the Dutch oven on top of the stove over a medium heat. Add the macadamia nut oil and onions. Cook until the onions are transparent. Remove the onions and set aside. Add the brisket to the pan and carefully brown on all sides. Top with the onions, celery, and peppers. Pour on the beef broth.

Place the brisket into the oven, with a lid that is slightly ajar, and bake for 3 1/2 hours or until tender. Remove the brisket from the oven and cool at room temperature for an hour. Take the meat out of the sauce, wrap it in parchment paper and then in aluminum foil, and refrigerate it. Refrigerate the sauce separately.

Half an hour before you are ready to serve, remove the brisket and the sauce from the refrigerator. Skim the fat from the top. Slice the meat and place it in a baking dish. Top with the sauce and bake at 350°F for 30 minutes.

Susan recommends freezing the brisket for a few days and then thawing, heating, and serving. She finds it is tastier that way.

Susan's Veal, Lamb, and Beef Stew

SERVES FOUR • **PHASES 1, 2, 3**

YOU WILL NEED: Heavy stockpot

2 tablespoons macadamia nut oil

1 1/2 pounds meat (1/2 pound each of veal, lamb, and beef or any combination—veal and lamb together give a wonderful flavor, cubed

1 tablespoon Beef Rub (page 65)

3 cloves garlic, minced

2 green peppers, diced

2 onions, diced

2 large stalks celery, diced

In a heavy stockpot, over a medium heat, brown the meat in the oil (about 2 minutes on each side. Add the herbs and vegetables. Mix well. Simmer for about 1 1/2 hours. Set aside to cool. Freeze leftovers in lunch-, snack-, and or dinner-sized servings. Reheat as desired.

Lamb-Stuffed Eggplant

SERVES FOUR • **PHASES 1, 2, 3**

YOU WILL NEED: Medium-sized pot
Medium-sized mixing bowl

6 baby eggplants or 1 small regular-sized globe eggplant
6 teaspoons extra virgin olive oil
1 1/2 pounds lamb, ground
3 teaspoons fresh rosemary (about 3 sprigs), minced
1/2 teaspoon sea salt

Preheat the oven to 350°F. Parboil the whole eggplant for about 10 minutes. Remove with a slotted spoon and let drain. When cool, halve the eggplant lengthwise and scoop out the pulp (keeping the skin intact). Chop the pulp with the olive oil. Combine the lamb, rosemary, and salt. Mix well. Add the eggplant pulp to the lamb and gently stuff the mixture into the eggplant shells. Bake at 350° for 30 minutes.

Roast Pork

SERVES SIX • **PHASES 1, 2, 3**

YOU WILL NEED: Roasting pan large enough to fit meat

4 to 5 pounds pork roast (preferably organic)
2 large cloves garlic, minced
1 tablespoon Seasoning Mix or Rub of your choice (pages 62–65)

Preheat the oven to 350°F. Wipe the meat with a damp cloth. Cut off any surplus fat and the edges of the roast. Rub well with garlic and seasoning mix. Place the meat fat side up in a roasting pan. Roast for 45 minutes per pound. The cooked meat will be grayish white. Keep the leftovers to eat as a snack.

Baby Lamb Chops

SERVES FOUR • **PHASES 1, 2, 3**

YOU WILL NEED: Small baking dish

4 teaspoons of your favorite Seasoning Mix (the Beef Rub on page 65 is ideal) for each lamb chop

4 baby lamb chops

4 teaspoons coconut butter

Preheat oven to 400°F. Press the herb rub into the lamb chop. Place it in a small baking dish. Top with the coconut butter. Bake for 10 minutes.

Three-Meat Meatloaf

SERVES SIX • **PHASES 2, 3**

YOU WILL NEED: Small skillet • Medium-sized mixing bowl • Loaf pan

2 tablespoons extra virgin olive oil

1 medium onion, diced

1/2 cup shallots, diced

3/4 pound veal, ground

3/4 pound lamb, ground

2 links turkey sausage, squeezed out of the casing

3 eggs

1 tablespoon Beef Rub (page 65)

1/2 pound herbed goat cheese, cut in 1/2-inch chunks

Preheat the oven to 350°F. Heat the oil in a skillet over medium-high heat. Add the onion and shallots. Sauté until browned.

Combine the sautéed onions and shallots with the veal, lamb, sausage, eggs, and Beef Rub together in the mixing bowl. Mix in the cheese.

Place the mixture in a loaf pan and bake at 350°F for 1 hour, 15 minutes. Allow to set 15 minutes before slicing.

MAIN DISHES: FISH

Baked Flounder in Parchment Paper

SERVES FOUR • **PHASES 1, 2, 3**

YOU WILL NEED: Parchment paper
Baking dish large enough to hold fish

2 medium flounder, filleted
1 large onion, diced
4 cloves garlic, minced
3 tablespoons sesame oil
2 teaspoons fresh tarragon, minced

Preheat the oven to 300°F. Wash and pat dry the fish. Put the parchment paper in the baking dish and place the fish in the center. Top the fish with the diced onion and garlic, and sprinkle with the sesame oil and tarragon. Bake for 30 minutes.

Roasted Shrimp

SERVES FOUR • **PHASES 1, 2, 3**

YOU WILL NEED: Sheet pan

1 pound large shrimp (preferably wild), shelled and deveined
Sesame oil
Herbes de Provence (page 63) to taste
1/2 teaspoon fresh garlic, minced

Preheat the oven to 400°F. Place the shrimp on a sheet pan, drizzle with the oil, and sprinkle with the Herbes de Provence and garlic. Toss to combine and spread the shrimp out in a single layer. Roast for 5 to 6 minutes, until the shrimp are cooked through. Don't overcook!

Coconut Scallops and Sugar Snap Peas

SERVES FOUR • **PHASES 1, 2, 3**

YOU WILL NEED: Wok or heavy fry pan

6 tablespoons coconut oil

2 cups sugar snap peas, washed and dried

2 pounds bay or sea scallops, washed and patted dry

1 teaspoon fresh ginger, peeled and grated

French or Celtic sea salt

Place 3 tablespoons of the coconut oil in a wok or heavy fry pan. Heat until very hot. Add the sugar snap peas, ginger, and pinch of salt. Stir-fry for 3 minutes, tossing often. Remove the peas and keep warm. Place the remaining tablespoon of oil into the wok. Add the scallops, remaining ginger, and additional salt to taste. Stir-fry for 5 minutes, just lightly browning the scallops. Toss the scallops and peapods together and serve hot.

Gingered Salmon

Quick and easy with gourmet flavors

SERVES SIX • **PHASES 2, 3**

YOU WILL NEED:
Baking dish large enough to hold fish

3 pounds fresh salmon

2 tablespoons olive oil

6 to 8 cloves garlic, minced

2 tablespoons fresh ginger, peeled and minced

1/2 cup fresh lemon juice

1/2 cup pecans, coarsely chopped

Preheat the oven to 350°F. Wash and pat dry the salmon. Place the fish in a baking dish. Brush the salmon with the olive oil and sprinkle with the garlic and ginger. Drizzle the lemon juice over the fish. Bake for 20 minutes. Remove the pan from the oven, top with the chopped pecans and serve warm.

Elegant Fish Rolls

Treat yourself to the best

SERVES SIX • **PHASES 2, 3**

YOU WILL NEED:
Baking dish large enough to hold six fish rolls
Food processor

6 small orange roughy fillets or other mild-flavored white fish

Juice of 1 lemon

French or Celtic sea salt to taste

3 tablespoons coconut butter, melted

1/2 cup macadamia nuts

One recipe of Spicy, Spicy, Spicy Crab Cakes (page 82)

Preheat the oven 450°F. Wash and pat dry the fish fillets. Sprinkle the fillets with lemon juice and salt, then brush them with the coconut butter.

Roughly chop the macadamia nuts in a food processor. Press the fillets into the crushed nuts. Place a heaping tablespoon of the crabmeat mixture in the center of each fish fillet, and fold the ends into the center to form a roll. Place the fillets in a baking dish. Bake for 20 minutes. Baste with the pan juices before serving.

Crunchy Salmon Florentine

SERVES FOUR • **PHASES 2, 3**

YOU WILL NEED:

Stainless steel fish poacher or glass baking dish with cover
Medium-sized non-stick skillet • Small non-stick skillet

1 large clove garlic, crushed

2 pounds fresh salmon

1/2 cup Fish Stock (page 77) or clam juice

1/2 cup lemon water (water mixed with juice of 1/2 lemon)

4 tablespoons Clarified Butter (page 66)

4 tablespoons sweet onion (like Vidalia), chopped

1/2 cup Garlic Walnuts (page 84), chopped

1 cup fresh spinach, stems removed, washed well and dried

Herbamare to taste

1/2 cup unsweetened coconut, shredded

Preheat the oven to 300°F. Spread the garlic on the salmon. Place the salmon on a poaching rack in a fish poacher. . Pour the fish stock and lemon water over the fish. Cover. Place the pan in the oven and allow the fish to poach for 20 minutes.

Melt 2 tablespoons of butter in a medium-sized skillet. Add the onion and sauté until transparent. Toss in the walnuts and dry spinach. Keep tossing until the spinach wilts (do not overcook). Season with some Herbamare. Remove to a warm dish.

Melt the remaining butter in a small non-stick skillet. Add the coconut and sauté until it begins to brown. Place the coconut on a paper towel to drain.

Remove the salmon from the poaching liquid and place on top of the spinach. Garnish with the coconut. Serve immediately.

Baked Trout with Apricot Sauce

SERVES FOUR • **PHASE 3**

YOU WILL NEED:
Baking pan large enough to hold fish
Small saucepan • Blender or food processor

2 pounds whole fresh trout, cleaned

1/2 cup fresh parsley on the stem

2 organic lemons, 1 cut into wedges, the other juiced and peel grated

1 organic lime, juiced and peel grated

1/2 cup water

2 teaspoons arrowroot powder

3 fresh apricots, pitted and chopped

1 tablespoon xylitol

1/2 cup fresh mint leaves

1 teaspoon Herbamare

1/3 cup macadamia nuts, chopped

Preheat the oven to 400°F. Place the trout in a baking pan. Place the parsley and the wedges from one lemon into the belly of the fish. Bake for 18 minutes.

Meanwhile place the lemon and lime juices, and their grated peels, into a saucepan. Add the water, arrowroot powder, and two-thirds of the chopped apricots. Simmer the sauce over medium heat, stirring, until thick.

Puree the apricot mixture in the blender with the xylitol, mint leaves, and Herbamare.

Place the fish on a platter and top with the sauce, macadamia nuts, and reserved chopped apricots.

Tuna with Plum Sauce

SERVES FOUR • **PHASE 3**

YOU WILL NEED: Non-stick grill
Small saucepan • Blender or food processor

4 serving-size tuna steaks

4 plums, pitted

1/2 cup grapefruit juice

1/2 cup water

Xylitol to taste, depending on sweetness of plums

1 tablespoon garlic or Finger-Lickin' Good Roasted Garlic (page 81), minced

1/2 teaspoon sea salt

Pinch white pepper

1/3 cup macadamia nuts, coarsely chopped

2 tablespoons scallions, sliced

Grill the tuna steaks the way you like them done.

Cook the plums in a saucepan over a medium heat with the grapefruit juice, water, xylitol (if needed), garlic, and salt and pepper. Cook until the plums are soft.

Puree the cooked plum mixture in a blender.

Place the tuna on serving platter. Spoon on the sauce. Top with the chopped macadamia nuts and scallions.

MAIN DISHES: POULTRY

Fabulous Roast Chicken

A small turkey can be prepared this same way

SERVES FOUR • **PHASES 1, 2, 3**

YOU WILL NEED:
Roasting pan • Parchment paper

2 pounds organic roasting chicken

Seasoned Salt (page 62) or Herbamare

2 gloves of garlic, minced

1/4 pound Clarified Butter (page 66), room temperature

Sprinkle the salt and garlic on the chicken inside and out. Allow it to sit for at least an hour.

Preheat the oven to 450°F. Rub the butter on the chicken making a thick coating. Sprinkle with more salt. Place the chicken in a baking pan that has been lined with large strips of parchment paper (or place in a clay pot). Wrap paper around the chicken so no steam can escape. Bake for 1 hour. Then turn the oven down to 325°F and let it bake for an hour more (or until tender). If you want the chicken to brown, remove the parchment paper the last 1/2 hour.

Chicken (or Turkey) Cakes

SERVES TWO • **PHASES 1, 2, 3**

YOU WILL NEED: Medium-sized bowl
Small fry pan • Small baking dish

1 1/2 cups organic chicken or turkey meat, ground

2 egg whites, beaten to soft peaks

1 teaspoon Poultry Rub (page 64)

Pinch of French or Celtic sea salt

Coconut oil for frying

2 tablespoons onion, chopped

2 large cloves garlic, minced

1/2 zucchini, shredded

1 tablespoon Clarified Butter (page 66)

1 recipe Hollandaise (page 68)
or Lemon Barbecue Sauce (page 65)

Preheat the oven to 375°F. Mix the poultry, egg whites, Poultry Rub, and salt in a bowl. Form into four balls that you flatten with the palm of your hand. Put enough coconut oil in a fry pan to cover generously. When it is hot, fry the patties in the coconut oil until crisp (about 3 minutes on each side), turning once.

Sauté the onions, garlic, and zucchini in the butter until the onions are lightly browned. Place the vegetable mixture in the baking dish with the browned cakes placed on the top.

Pour the sauce of your choice over the top. Bake for 10 minutes.

Lemon Chicken

SERVES FOUR • **PHASES 1, 2, 3**

YOU WILL NEED: Roasting pan

2 pounds organic chicken, cut into eight pieces

1 teaspoon fresh oregano, minced

2 cloves garlic, minced

1/4 cup Clarified Butter (page 66)

Herbamare

Juice of 2 lemons

Preheat the oven 400°F. Rub the chicken with oregano and garlic. Melt the butter in a roasting pan. Roll the chicken pieces in the butter. Sprinkle with Herbamare.

Roast the chicken, skin side up and uncovered for 30 minutes or until golden brown. Turn the pieces over and continue roasting and browning for another 30 minutes. Reduce the heat to 300°F and continue to cook until tender.

Squeeze the lemon juice over the chicken. Cover and allow it to sit in a turned-off oven for 15 minutes before serving.

Raspberry Duck

SERVES FOUR • **PHASE 3**

YOU WILL NEED: Small saucepan
Deep roasting pan with a rack • Baster or ladle
Gravy separator • Blender or food processor
Small sharp pointed knife

4 pounds duck

1 1/2 pounds fresh raspberries
(save 10 for garnish)

1 bunch fresh tarragon stalks
(save 6 1-inch tips for garnish)

1 large onion

1 tablespoon Poultry Rub (page 64)

3 tablespoons almond butter

Salt and pepper

Preheat the oven to 325°F. Separate the skin from the meat on each side of the duck breast, forming two pockets. (A small pointed sharp knife will do this job.) Do not break the skin. Insert 1 dozen of the raspberries, and 2 stalks of the tarragon into each of the pockets. Secure the onion and remaining tarragon stalks in the cavity of the duck. Salt and pepper the duck's skin.

Place the duck onto the rack of a small roasting pan. Bake for 3 1/2 hours. As the duck bakes, it renders about 1 quart of fat. Remove the accumulating fat with a baster or ladle about every half hour. When the duck is cooked, the skin will be brown and crisp. Separate the cooking juices with a gravy separator.

Remove the onion from the duck's cavity. Place it in a blender with the duck-renderings (that you have just separated from the fat) and puree it. Pour the pureed mixture into a saucepan. Add the almond butter, mix well, and simmer until the mixture thickens.

Slice the duck meat onto a warm platter. Spoon the sauce over the meat. Garnish with raspberries and tarragon tips.

COOKIES AND SORBETS

Chinese-Almond Cookies

MAKES 16 WALNUT-SIZED COOKIES • **PHASES 2, 3**

YOU WILL NEED: Food processor
Medium-sized mixing bowl • Electric mixer
Small bowl of cold water
Large cookie sheet lined with parchment paper
Cooling rack

1/4 cup unsalted ground almonds
1/4 cup natural, smooth almond butter
1/3 cup goat cream cheese, room temperature
1 teaspoon almond extract
1/2 teaspoon vanilla extract
2 tablespoons xylitol
2 tablespoons whey protein (vanilla bean flavor)
1/2 teaspoon baking powder
1/2 tablespoon sliced almonds (16 slices)

Preheat the oven to 375°F. Place all of the ingredients, except the almond slices, into the bowl of an electric mixer in the order listed. Blend well after each addition. Beat at a medium speed until well blended.

Dip your fingers in cold water, and roll the dough into walnut-sized balls. Carefully place the ball on a cookie sheet lined with parchment paper. Place a slivered almond in the center of each cookie. Place the cookies in the oven and bake for 10 minutes. Remove the cookies to a cooling rack, and allow them to cool completely before eating.

Coconut-Pecan Wows

MAKES 16 WALNUT-SIZED COOKIES • **PHASES 2, 3**

***YOU WILL NEED:* Food processor**
Medium-sized mixing bowl • Electric mixer
Bowl of cold water
Large cookie sheet lined with parchment paper
Cooling rack

1/3 cup unsalted ground pecans

1/3 cup unsweetened coconut

1/3 cup goat cream cheese, room temperature

1 teaspoon vanilla

2 tablespoons xylitol

1 tablespoon whey protein (vanilla bean flavor)

1/2 teaspoon baking powder

2 tablespoons pecans (16 halves)

Preheat the oven to 375°F. Place all of the ingredients, except the pecan halves, into the bowl of an electric mixer in the order listed. Beat at a medium speed after each addition until well blended.

Wet your fingers with the cold water. Roll the dough into walnut-sized balls and place the balls on a cookie sheet lined with parchment paper. Press a pecan half into the center of each cookie. Put the cookies in the oven and bake for10 minutes. Remove the cookies to a rack and allow them to cool before eating.

Peanut Butter Cookies

MAKES 16 COOKIES • **PHASES 2, 3**

YOU WILL NEED: Food processor
Medium-sized mixing bowl • Electric mixer
Large cookie sheet lined with parchment paper
Cooling rack

1/4 cup unsalted ground peanuts

1/4 cup smooth, natural peanut butter (without added sugar)

1/3 cup goat cream cheese, room temperature

1 teaspoon vanilla

2 tablespoons xylitol

1 tablespoon whey protein (vanilla bean flavor)

1/2 teaspoon baking powder

2 teaspoons peanuts (16 peanut halves)

Preheat the oven to 375°F. Place all of the ingredients, except the peanut halves, into the bowl of an electric mixer in the order listed. Beat at a medium speed after each addition until well blended.

Roll the dough into walnut-sized balls and place on a cookie sheet lined with parchment paper. Gently press half a peanut in the center of each cookie. Place the cookies in the oven and bake for 10 minutes. Remove the cookies to a rack and allow them to cool before eating.

Love-These-Meringue Cookies

MAKES 20 COOKIES • **PHASES 2, 3**

YOU WILL NEED:
Electric mixer • Food processor
Large cookie sheet lined with parchment paper

2 egg whites, room temperature

1/2 teaspoon cream of tartar

1/4 teaspoon salt

2/3 cup xylitol

3/4 cup walnuts, chopped in food processor

Preheat the oven to 275°F. Place the egg whites, cream of tartar, salt, and xylitol in the smallest bowl of your electric mixer. Beat until the whites are stiff. Carefully fold the chopped walnuts into the stiff egg whites using a rubber spatula. Do not break down the stiffness of the egg whites.

Drop the cookies by teaspoonfuls onto a cookie sheet lined with parchment paper. Set them 1-inch apart. Place the cookies in the oven and bake for 20 minutes (or until they begin to brown.) Turn the oven off, and leave cookies in the oven to crisp overnight. They will melt in your mouth.

Blueberry Sorbet

MAKES SIX $^1/_2$-CUP SERVINGS • **PHASE 3**

*YOU WILL NEED: **Blender or food processor***
Ice cream maker or ice cube trays

$2^1/_2$ cups fresh blueberries

$^3/_4$ cup xylitol

$^1/_2$ cup water

$^1/_2$ cup goat yogurt

Puree the blueberries, xylitol, water, and yogurt in a blender. Pour the mixture into an ice cream maker, and freeze according to manufacturer's directions. Scoop out the sorbet with a ball scoop. The sorbet may also be frozen in ice cube trays.

Cantaloupe Sorbet

MAKES SIX $^1/_2$-CUP SERVINGS • **PHASE 3**

*YOU WILL NEED: **Blender or food processor***
Medium-sized mixing bowl
Ice cream maker or ice cube trays

2 cups ripe cantaloupe,
peeled and pureed

$^3/_4$ cup xylitol

$^3/_4$ cup water

2 tablespoons fresh ginger,
peeled and grated

Using a knife, separate the cantaloupe skin from its flesh. Puree the fruit in a in a blender. Whisk together the cantaloupe puree, xylitol, water, and ginger in a mixing bowl. Pour the mixture into an ice cream maker, and freeze according to manufacturer's directions. The sorbet can also be frozen in ice cube trays.

MEAL PLANS

Meal plans can be your best friend when it comes to changing the way you eat. They can organize your thinking and make it easier to shop for foods that are healthiest for your body, and they can challenge your imagination and inspire you to create meals you will truly enjoy eating.

I suggest that you make the Seasoning Mixes (pages 62–65) that you like, and then freeze them. They can turn a simple omelet or burger into a special meal.

Make the Clarified Butter (page 66) so you have that easily accessible in the refrigerator.

I also like to keep the Ginger Lemonade (page 72) on hand. Drink it each morning for breakfast. It lasts a long time in the refrigerator, tastes good, and is great for digestion. Drink it hot or cold throughout the day or alternate it with water and fresh lemon.

The following five-day meal plans are an example of how you can eat deliciously on Dr. Levin's Yeast-Free Diet. We do not expect you to follow these plans "to the letter," rather use them as general recommendations and suggestions for eating.

There are no restrictions on portions. Use common sense and eat until you feel full.

PHASE 1 MEAL PLANS

Day 1

Breakfast
Tasty Egg Pancakes, 72
Ginger Lemonade, 72

Mid-morning snack
Celery and cucumber slices with Susan's Yeast-Free Salad Dressing, 67

Lunch
Green Bean Salad (page 98) with your choice of leftover meat, fish, or poultry

Afternoon snack
Coconut Scallops and Sugar Snap Peas, 109

Dinner
Roast Pork, 106
Oven-Roasted Vegetables, 93

Day 2

Breakfast
Chicken (or Turkey) Cakes (page 115) topped with a poached egg
Ginger Lemonade, 72

Mid-morning snack
Rich Chicken Stock (page 79) or store-bought, organic, sugar-free chicken broth with Soup Noodles, 89

Lunch
Your favorite lettuce tossed with cucumbers and radishes, topped with leftover pork and Lemon Barbecue Sauce, 65

Afternoon snack
Oven-Roasted Vegetables (page 93) leftover from Day 1

Dinner
Susan's Veal, Lamb, and Beef Stew, 105
Steamed broccoli with Clarified Butter (page 66) and your favorite Seasoning Mix, 62–65

Day 3

Breakfast
Sunny-side-up eggs with organic chicken sausage
Ginger Lemonade, 72

Mid-morning snack
Latkas, 94

Lunch
Garlic Soup (page 89) and leftover Coconut Scallops and Sugar Pea Pods, 109

Afternoon snack

Roast beef slices sprinkled with Beef Rub (page 65) and topped with Lemon Barbecue Sauce (page 65), then rolled up

Dinner

Lamb-Stuffed Eggplant, 106
Zucchini sautéed in olive oil

Day 4

Breakfast

Sweet Fritters, 71
Ginger Lemonade, 72

Mid-morning snack

Medley of raw vegetables sprinkled with Herbamare

Lunch

Leftovers from Susan's Veal, Lamb, and Beef Stew from Day 2
Green salad with Susan's Yeast-Free Salad Dressing, 67

Afternoon snack

Turkey with Mustard-Dill Sauce, 69

Dinner

The Levin's Chicken Soup (page 88) with Soup Noodles, 89
Spaghetti the Squash Way, 94

Day 5

Breakfast

Deviled Salmon Eggs, 71
Ginger Lemonade, 72

Mid-morning snack

Leftover chicken used to make soup from Day 4 with Hollandaise, 68

Lunch

Roasted Shrimp (page 108) with Lemon Barbecue Sauce (page 65) on a bed of lettuce

Afternoon snack

Finger-Lickin' Good Roasted Garlic (page 81) spread on celery stalks

Dinner

Baby Lamb Chops (page 107) with a steamed vegetable of your choice

PHASE 2 MEAL PLANS

You may want to try making the Popovers (page 73). They are a delicious bread substitute to have on hand; you can even make an elegant sandwich with them. And don't forget to check out the cookies!

Day 1

Breakfast
Scrambled eggs, onions, and goat cream cheese
Ginger Lemonade, 72

Mid-morning snack
Garlic Walnuts, 84

Lunch
Gently Flavored Cauliflower Soup, 90
Roasted Shrimp, 108

Afternoon snack
Peanut Butter Cookies, 120

Dinner
Crabby, Crabby, Crabby Crab Cakes, 81
Zucchini in Sweet Peanut Sauce, 96

Day Two

Breakfast
Deviled Salmon Eggs, 71
Popover (page 73) with goat cream cheese
Ginger Lemonade, 72

Mid-morning snack
Sliced cucumbers and Susan's Yeast-Free Salad Dressing, 67

Lunch
Favorite Chicken Salad (page 100) on a bed of lettuce

Afternoon snack
Coconut-Pecan Wows, 119

Dinner
Brisket of Beef (page 104) over Soup Noodles, 89
Steamed broccoli topped with toasted pine nuts

Day 3

Breakfast
Tasty Egg Pancakes, 72
Ginger Lemonade, 72

Mid-morning snack
Sweet Pecans, 84

Lunch
Vermont Salad, 100

Afternoon snack

Leftover Chicken Salad from Phase 1, Day 2

Dinner

Salmon Chowder, 91
Asparagus Gone Nuts, 95

Day 4

Breakfast

Basic Omelet (page 70) with herbed goat cheese

Mid-morning snack

Spicy Almonds, 86

Lunch

Leftover Salmon Chowder from Day 3

Afternoon snack

Boiled or sautéed shrimp with Thousand Island Dressing, 101

Dinner

Raspberry Duck (page 117) with Crunchy Bok Choy, 96

Day 5

Breakfast

Leftover duck from Day 4 and scrambled eggs

Mid-morning snack

1 dozen nuts of your choice

Lunch

Split Pea Soup, 92
Popover (page 73) with boiled ham and Thousand Island Dressing, 101

Afternoon snack

Leftover Lamb from Phase 1, Day 5 with Mustard-Dill Sauce, 69

Dinner

So You Think You Can't Eat Pizza, 85
Zucchini in Sweet Peanut Sauce, 96

PHASE 3 MEAL PLANS

This phase adds low-carbohydrate fruits. It is a very healthy and livable diet plan to follow for a lifetime.

Day 1

Breakfast
Sausage Frittata, 74
Ginger Lemonade, 72

Mid-morning snack
Garlic Walnuts, 84

Lunch
Chicken (or Turkey) Cakes, 115

Afternoon snack
Chinese Almond Cookies, 118

Dinner
Lamb-Stuffed Eggplant, 106

Day 2

Breakfast
Fresh Raspberry Omelet, 75

Mid-morning snack
Sweet Pecans, 84

Lunch
Coconut Shrimp with Peach Sauce, 87

Afternoon snack
Love-These-Meringue Cookies, 121

Dinner
Elegant Fish Rolls, 110
Snow pea pods raw or sautéed in sesame oil

Day 3

Breakfast
Ginger, Pumpkin Seed, and Swiss-Surprise Omelet, 76
Ginger Lemonade, 72

Mid-morning snack
Caponata, 97

Lunch
Turkey slices filled with herbed goat cheese and chopped scallions and rolled, topped with Thousand Island Dressing, 101

Afternoon snack
Sweet Pecans, 84

Dinner
Tuna with Plum Sauce, 113
Brussels sprouts mixed with Finger-Lickin' Good Roasted Garlic, 81

Day 4

Breakfast
Sweet Fritters, 71
Ginger Lemonade, 72

Mid-morning snacks
Spicy Almonds, 86

Lunch
Crabby, Crabby, Crabby Crab Cakes (page 81) on lettuce leaves

Afternoon snack
Parmesan Crackers, 86

Dinner
Crunchy Salmon Florentine, 111
Steamed or sautéed patty pan squash
Chinese Almond Cookies, 118

Day 5

Breakfast
Fried steak and eggs
Ginger Lemonade, 72

Mid-morning snack
Sweet Pecans, 84

Lunch
Mixed lettuces and cut vegetables topped with leftover salmon from Day 4 and Lemon Barbecue Sauce, 65

Afternoon snack
Peanut Butter Cookies, 120

Dinner
Three-Meat Meatloaf, 107
Blueberry Sorbet, 122

7 Dining Out

with Susan Levin

At this point you may be wondering, is it possible to eat out on Dr. Levin's Yeast-Free Diet? Susan, Dr. Levin's wife and the go-to person in his practice and his life, has been asked this question so often from patients that she asked to include a chapter on it. In short, the answer to that question is yes—just order carefully. Most restaurants have become much more health conscious and are happy to cook your food to order.

TYPES OF CUISINE

Different types of cuisines will pose different types of challenges. For guidelines on how on to overcome these challenges when eating specific cuisines, read on. Not all cuisines are included, but you will get the general idea of what you can eat when dining in a restaurant. If you are in doubt, please don't be afraid to ask about the ingredients in the dishes. Say, "I am on a special diet for my health and cannot eat many foods. Can you please tell me exactly what is in this dish?" You will be pleasantly surprised to find that most restaurants are accustomed to these questions, and are very helpful.

Chinese Restaurants

A number of different styles contribute to Chinese cuisine, but perhaps the best known and most influential are Cantonese cuisine, Shandong cuisine, Jiangsu cuisine, and Szechuan cuisine. One style may favor the use of lots of garlic and shallots over lots of chilies and spices, while another may favor preparing seafood over other meats and fowl. One cuisine may favor cooking techniques such as braising and stewing, while another cuisine employs baking and stir-frying. Many traditional regional cuisines rely on basic methods of preservation such as drying, salting, pickling, and fermentation. Chinese cuisine, at its best, is prepared with fresh fish but also includes great sources of protein from poultry, lamb, beef, chicken, and a wonderful assortment of vegetables (asparagus, baby cabbage, bok choy, broccoli, eggplant, onions, spinach, string beans, etc.), as well many spices including ginger and garlic. Thus, you have a wide variety of choices.

Watch out for sugar and monosodium glutamate (MSG) hidden in the sauces, soups, condiments and dips, as well as rice vinegars, soy sauce, Teriyaki sauce, and oyster sauce, which usually contain wheat, sugar, and cornstarch or other thickeners. Ask for sauces to be served on the side, or better yet not at all. If you love Chinese food you will enjoy it even more as you taste all the wonderful ingredients without a thick sauce to cover it up.

Steer clear of dishes with fermented soy and soy in any form. Soy is 100 percent genetically modified today, and unless it is organic, do not eat it. It is also best to avoid all fresh and dried mushroom and other fungi, noodle- and white-rice-based dishes, and any food that is deep-fried such as deep fried chicken or fish.

So what is left to eat? Choose dishes with steamed, grilled, or stir-fried fish, poultry, beef, lamb, or pork with vegetables, except for carrots, corn, green peas, and other high-carbohydrate (starchy) vegetables. Here are several safe suggestions:

- Moo Shu chicken, pork, or shrimp
- Roasted duck or sautéed beef
- Seafood combination

- Chicken lettuce wraps
- Chicken with cashew nuts (Phases 2, 3)
- Eggplant or lamb with garlic sauce (Phases 2, 3)
- Brown rice and vegetables with pork (Phase 3)
- Seared fish with black bean sauce (Phase 3)

Remember, once you arrive at Phase 3 you still need to ask for a list of ingredients, and always stay away from cornstarch, sugar, white rice, thickeners, MSG and soy! Most Chinese restaurants are more than happy to substitute different choices of proteins even if they're not on the menu. So if you prefer chicken, seafood, or pork, don't hesitate to ask for it. If nothing looks appropriate, you can always order a protein with steamed or stir-fried vegetables. Enjoy your meal with a cup of green tea.

French Restaurants

Classic French food, or haute cuisine (meaning high cooking), typically involves elaborately prepared dishes made with rich sauces and other gourmet ingredients. Nonetheless, there are not too many challenges in this kind of cuisine. Common sense should prevail, but fine French food includes just about everything that can be eaten be it in Phase 1 to Phase 3. The French love fresh ingredients.

In the initial stages of the diet, the challenges are in the wine used for cooking, creams, mushrooms, and starchy vegetables such as carrots, corn, and green peas. Boiled new potatoes have one of the highest carbohydrate counts, so please abstain. As always, check your ingredients. There is so much to eat and enjoy.

- Baked or poached salmon, or salmon en papillote
- Escargots in butter and garlic
- Dover sole with lemon butter
- Asparagus with hollandaise sauce (Phases 2, 3)

- Calves liver (Phases 2, 3)
- Foie gras (Phases 2, 3)
- Lobster bisque (Phase 3)
- Ratatouille (Phase 3)

Desserts are hard to say no to, but try to have some fresh berries or melon if in Phase 3. And you can always splurge and add cream in Phase 3 to your berries. Decaf latte with cream is a wonderful choice as is decaf espresso.

German Restaurants

In authentic German cuisine, meat, especially pork, veal, game, and sausage (of which there are over 1,500 types), potatoes, sauerkraut (fermented cabbage), wheat, rye, and fats of animal origin predominate. Foods tend to be boiled, steamed, or deep-fried, often prepared with breadcrumbs and served with rich gravies thickened with heavy cream and starch. Vegetables are used most often used in stews and soups. Carrots, turnips, spinach, peas, beans, broccoli, and many types of cabbage are very common. German dishes are rarely hot and spicy. Popular herbs include parsley, thyme, laurel, chives, black pepper (used in small amounts), juniper berries, and caraway. Cardamom, anise seed, and cinnamon are often used. Horseradish is considered a favorite in German cuisine.

While German restaurants pose the greatest challenge during Phase 1 for those hoping to enjoy classic German dishes such as weiner schnitzel (breaded, deep-fried veal) and spaetzle (egg noodles), more choices become available in Phases 2 and 3. Always check whether flour or breadcrumbs, as well as sugar, cream, potatoes, and starch are added before ordering any of the dishes below. If in doubt, you can always ask for a broiled meat or fish.

- German meatloaf
- Spargel (white asparagus)
- Steak tartare

- Poached trout
- Roasted pork
- Cabbage rolls (Phases 2, 3)
- Kielbasa (Phases 2, 3, if prepared without sugar)
- German meatballs (Phases 2, 3)

Indian Restaurants

Vegetables are an integral part of Indian cuisine as vegetarianism is practiced in much of India. Legumes such as chickpeas and lentils, rice, wheat, spices, herbs, vegetables, and fruits are at the heart of much of India's cuisine. Turmeric, garam marsala, cumin, and coriander are used to season many Indian stews and their coconut- and yogurt-based based curries and sauces. Non-vegetarian dishes are mainly comprised of eggs, seafood, lamb, and chicken.

Despite Indian cuisine's reliance on ingredients that are eliminated in the early phases of Dr. Levin's Yeast-Free Diet, look for dishes that are simply prepared. Watch out for cornstarch, sugar, and wheat flour in many Indian pastes, chutneys, curries, and sauces. Many of the curries and sauces also tend to contain creams and lots of seasonings and yogurt. Check your ingredients and in Phase 3, a dish with yogurt or that is moderately spiced might work.

- Vegetable kebabs
- Lamb or chicken kebabs
- Chicken with cashew nuts (Phases 2, 3)
- Shrimp with lentils (Phases 2, 3)
- Split pea dhal (Phase 3)
- Eggplant with tomato sauce (Phase 3)
- Tandoori chicken (Phase 3)
- Curried lentil and chickpea stew (Phase 3)

Italian Restaurants

Italian restaurants are commonplace everywhere in the city or suburbs and easily outnumber any other cuisine—except American fast food. While Italian food isn't simplistic cuisine, it can be prepared simply with olive oil, lemon, garlic and fresh herbs—ingredients that are acceptable in all three phases of Dr. Levin's Yeast-Free Diet. And while many pastas, polentas, and risottos will initially be off-limits, the Italian's simple preparation of meats, poultry, and seafood, and a variety of fresh vegetable and bean dishes can make for some delicious meals.

The greatest challenge is to avoid pasta dishes and those with olives, capers, tomatoes, and aged cheeses. Steer clear of Parmesan (an aged cheese) and opt for low-carbohydrate fresh cheeses such as goat and sheep cheese, mozzarella, and ricotta in the later phases of the diet. And, sorry, abstain from the bread. Yams and brown rice in limited portions are allowed in Phase 3 but be judicious.

- Grilled or broiled lamb, beef, pork, poultry, or steak
- Grilled fish, shrimp, or chicken breast
- Sauté of mixed greens or broccoli rabe
- Vegetable frittata
- Spinach salad (without bacon and croutons)
- Mozzarella, tomato, and basil salad (Phase 3)
- Grilled fish with green beans, tomatoes, and basil (Phase 3)
- Seafood sauté in garlic-white wine* or marinara sauce (Phase 3)
- Osso buco* (Phase 3)

If you are in Phase 3, top off your dessert with an organic tea or decaf latte or espresso served with cream.

*Note: While wine and alcohol are eliminated on Dr. Levin's Yeast-Free Diet, the use of wine is acceptable when cooked because the alcohol evaporates.

Japanese Restaurants

Eating out at a Japanese restaurant during Phases 1 and 2 is somewhat challenging. Seafood, vegetables, and rice are mainstays in Japanese cuisine. Food preparation relies heavily on deep-frying, sweetened sauces, pickled foods, and fermented flavorings like soy or teriyaki sauce, and miso.

The best food in this situation would be any kind of sashimi (thinly sliced, raw seafood), as well as any of the dishes below. Be sure to omit dishes with rice in Phases 1 and 2, and order brown rice only in Phase 3. Avoid deep-fried dishes, such as tempura, and items with wasabi, miso, and other condiments. Steer clear of all soyfoods and soyfood products, including tofu, soybeans, soy sauce, and edamame, and avoid mushrooms and other fungi.

Enjoy while sipping a cup of green or herbal tea.

- Broiled fish, seafood, beef, or chicken
- Vegetable roll with cucumber, avocado, and asparagus
- Salmon roll (depending on ingredients)
- Sesame-ginger salmon
- Seared tuna with sesame
- Yosenabe with seafood and vegetables in clear broth (Phases 2, 3)
- Vegetables and brown rice (Phase 3)
- Grilled salmon with vegetables and soba noodles (Phase 3)

Mexican Restaurants

Mexican cuisine is actually a fusion of indigenous Mesoamerican cooking with European, especially Spanish, cooking developed after the Spanish conquest of the Aztec Empire. However, to this day, the basic staples remain the native beans, corn, chili peppers, and rice. Many traditional Mexican dishes from tacos and enchiladas to tamales and burritos are loaded with cheese, sour cream, and meat that have been prepared with lard.

Choose dishes such as burritos, enchiladas and tacos menu items with vegetables and mahi-mahi, chicken, ground turkey, crabmeat or shrimp, or meat that has been baked, broiled, or grilled. In Phases 2, 3, you may add some delicious pinto or black beans sprinkled with queso fresco, and in Phase 3 some tomatoes and rice. It is best to refrain from eating both beans and rice, which are high in carbohydrates. Instead opt for one or the other. Check the ingredients of sauces for additives and thickeners. If you like cilantro it is a wonderful seasoning and adds great flavor to dishes.

- Steak, chicken, or shrimp fajitas
- Carne asada (if prepared without sugar)
- Guacamole (Phases 2, 3)
- Seafood with pico de gallo and avocado-tomatillo salsa (Phases 2, 3)
- Vegetable salad with queso fresco (Phases 2, 3)
- Ceviche (Phases 2, 3)
- Beef soup served with brown rice (Phase 3)
- Chorizo with smothered vegetables (Phase 3)

In Phase 3, you may add some corn tortillas, but remember in this country corn is genetically modified. Best to eat only organic, but a treat now and then unless you have a corn allergy should be fine.

Middle Eastern Restaurants

Middle Eastern cuisine is a combination of the various countries and peoples of the Middle East and Western Asia. Some commonly used ingredients include olives and olive oil, pitas and flatbreads, lamb and chicken, honey, sesame seeds, dates, chickpeas, mint, and parsley.

Many spices are used in Middle Eastern food, particularly cumin, cinnamon, and clove, so ask before you bite! Kebabs of all varieties are a great way to eat in Middle Eastern restaurants. Chicken, beef, lamb, pork, and shrimp kebabs are served with vegetables and often rice. Avoid the rice until Phase 3, and refrain from eating it altogether unless it's brown rice. Middle Eastern restaurants usually offer a good variety of fish, so check out the fresh catch of the day, including many of the menu items below:

- Gyro (minus pita bread)
- Soulvakis (if prepared without sugar)
- Fried cauliflower or eggplant (Phases 2, 3)
- Bean fritters (Phases 2, 3)
- Baba ghanoush (Phases 2, 3)
- Tabbouleh (Phase 3)
- Fattousch (Phase 3)
- Tandoori chicken (Phase 3)

Tahini (sesame seed butter) is used in many Middle Eastern dishes. If it is freshly made, you may eat dishes containing it in Phases 2, 3. For a treat in Phase 3, try labneh, a traditional thick strained yogurt drink.

American Steak and Seafood Restaurants

Because American cuisine is as diverse as its population for our purposes here we'll focus on the popular seafood restaurants and steakhouses. In these types of restaurants it is relatively easy to control the types of ingredients used and how the dishes are prepared.

The range of fresh fish is endless. Snapper, salmon, halibut, cod, catfish, sole, flounder, grouper, halibut, herring, and mahi-mahi are among the many choices. Some fish are endangered and some are only available farm-raised. We recommend neither. Check with your server. Wild-caught fish will be the best and the healthiest. Most restaurants offer a fresh catch of the day. All kinds of fish can be sautéed, grilled, broiled, or poached. Fish should not be fried with breading or flour of any kind.

All cuts of red meat are acceptable, including fillet mignon, porterhouse steak, short ribs, strip steak, and more. Different cuts of meat can be cooked simply with fresh herbs and seasonings and grilled or broiled with a variety of vegetables. Skip the side order of French fries and consider some of these options:

- Shrimp cocktail
- Raw bar (clams and oysters)
- Skewered shrimp or beef kebabs
- Mussels or clams steamed in garlic and white wine* (Phases 2, 3)
- Mixed green salad with farmer's cheese (Phases 2, 3)
- Sweet potato fries (Phase 3)
- Spinach or Greek salad with olives (Phase 3)
- Grilled vegetable gazpacho (Phase 3)

*Note: While wine and alcohol are eliminated on Dr. Levin's Yeast-Free Diet, the use of wine is acceptable when cooked because the alcohol evaporates. In Phase 3, vodka and aquavit are allowed. Vodka is distilled and is not a grain, and aquavit (also called snaps) is distilled caraway seed.

Fast Food: On the Go

Chances are you are not going to have a choice of organic food at fast-food chains. However, some of these fast-food establishments are surprisingly open to trying to meet individual requests.

- Best bet at Subway (Phases 1, 2, and 3): Salad with vegetables, tuna, roasted chicken, or Black Forest ham. If some of the ingredients don't look fresh or are not acceptable on Dr. Levin's Yeast-Free Diet, ask the food preparer to eliminate them. Try lemon wedges for salad dressing, as the olive oil will not be the quality we feel you deserve and need.

- Best bet at diners (Phases 1, 2, and 3): Diners are abundant throughout the United States and are often a better choice than some of the other fast-food chains. You can get fresh eggs, steaks and chops, and even cooked vegetables. In many diners, you can ask them to use butter and not oil, as it is usually hydrogenated. Greek salads with feta (preferably from sheep or goat) are a common entrée at diners and are acceptable in Phase 2. Chef salads and Cobb salads are also popular. If dining out in Phase 2, ask to substitute the Swiss cheese in these salads for feta. Swiss cheese may be added in Phase 3. Please refrain from the mixed salad dressings.
- On the road or in the air (Phases 1, 2, and 3): When traveling by car or plane, you can always carry seasonings, spices, hard-boiled eggs, roast beef, turkey breast, Black Forest ham, and canned fish in oil from a variety of healthful food sources. Once you are allowed to have fruit, apples, pears, and berries are easy to carry. Most airlines are responsive to people with special diets and are often permit you to carry foods without irradiating them. So, once again, don't be afraid to ask.

IF IN DOUBT: GENERAL GUIDELINES TO DINE BY

In general, avoid all alcoholic beverages and have club soda or mineral water. Order broiled, grilled, or poached meat, chicken, fish, or other animal protein, and specify that no sugar, mushrooms, vinegar, or wheat be used in the preparation of any sauce. Fresh herbs and lemon are delicious alternatives to thick heavy sauces. Simple, plain items are obviously the safest choice, accompanied by steamed vegetables and a salad. Have oil and lemon juice on your salad. Skip the bread, crackers, and dessert.

If in doubt about the ingredients, always ask! And above all, enjoy.

PART THREE

Beyond Candida: Conditions Related to CRC

8 The Candida Connection

In this section, we will learn more about the patients that I introduced you to in the Patient Quiz, and in many cases, I will go beyond "beyond the yeast connection" to discuss some examples of how complicated CRC can become when left untreated.

Traditional medicine does not test for Candida and the unrecognized presentations of CRC are still not taught in medical schools or even in residency training programs. I will define CRC very broadly with case studies of patients who have come to me for maladies other than Candida infection and have had to address their CRC before their other health problems could be solved. Join me on a journey into the lives and health of some of my most representative CRC patients.

ACNE

Brianna came to see me in her late teens with severe facial acne and skin rashes bordering on psoriasis that had spread to her shoulders and anterior chest. Her face was devastatingly disturbing, even with heavy makeup. She had "tried everything," including seeing many dermatologists and having local evacuation of some of the larger cystic lesions, which always left scarring. She applied all sorts of topical creams and solutions of soaps and detergents, but to no avail. She had been on tetracycline antibiotics (a common treatment for severe acne) for over a year, and then more tetracycline for the repeated aggravations that followed when she stopped the antibiotics.

Brianna's Story

Brianna's doctors had not mentioned to her that the antibiotics were running roughshod over her intestinal flora. Not only were the antibiotics killing the bacteria responsible for the acne, they were also destroying the beneficial bacteria that normally help keep Candida levels in check. That was my first concern. I asked, "Did anyone check your stool"? She said, "No." I then asked, "Do you have a problem with vaginal infection"? She answered, "Yes, I have a white discharge all the time. It doesn't get better." This is an obvious diagnosis that had been missed by a school of the most prominent, well-respected physicians in New York.

I requested the usual stool analysis test, as well as a controversial procedure at that time called dark-field microscopic blood analysis. This technique uses a darkfield microscope to provide high contrast images and is able to detect the presence of immune disorders such as yeast infections in a drop of blood. A diagnosis of CRC was clear from the results.

Because Brianna's prior treatment had involved long-continuous antibiotic therapy, I treated her Candida infection aggressively with a combination of oral nystatin, the systemically absorbed antifungal Diflucan (fluconazole), and massive doses of probiotics. Needless to say, I also suggested Brianna strictly adhere to Phase 1 of my Yeast-Free Diet.

Shortly after beginning treatment, this young woman had a dramatic change in her life. Her lesions gradually started to reduce in size and severity, and their redness disappeared. She ended up a couple of years later with the typical scars of serious acne (the white depressions which indicate that terrible time in the past), and was able subsequently to have facial treatments and surgery so that she has ended up a beautiful woman with signs of her acne very difficult to see except on close examination.

CLINICAL PEARL: ACNE AND ALLERGY

One of the most common indications for long-term tetracycline therapy is acne that is resistant to treatment. When acne fails to respond to the antibiotics, it is frequently because the skin eruption is complicated by an allergic reaction to the Candida organism. Since the treatment prescribed was for long-term antibiotic therapy, not clearing the acne is frequently considered a problem of resistant bacteria. The traditional medical response is either to increase the dose or substitute another antibiotic, while the CRC complication goes unrecognized.

AUTISM AND LYME DISEASE

The rising incidence of autism is alarming and, in my opinion, is clearly related to the environmental changes that human beings have relentlessly heaped onto the "civilized" areas of our planet. These changes have now spread to the farthest reaches of the globe, creating challenges that must be faced, investigated, understood, and corrected, or human life as we know it will no longer be remembered, because no living thing will have enough brains to remember anything.

Shook's Story

Shook was a forty-year-old woman from India, married, with two children. One of her children had been diagnosed with pervasive developmental disorder (PDD), a form of autism spectrum disorder that involves delayed or impaired communication and social skills, behaviors, and learning skills. She said that her pregnancy and delivery were uneventful, and that the child developed normally until he was about fifteen months old, when he got his routine measles, mumps, and rubella (MMR) vaccination. Shortly afterward, he developed a fever and irritability, and gradually went into a health decline.

Before focusing on Shook's child, I asked whether she had any kind of prolonged antibiotic therapy before having the baby. She mentioned that she had been treated for sinusitis (inflammation of the lining of the sinuses), but that the antibiotic hadn't worked so she was given another antibiotic. Shook took the antibiotics for over a month. She felt that she had recovered from the respiratory problem. (Usually, sinusitis develops after an upper respiratory infection like the common cold.) When she became pregnant she noticed a white discharge with itching from her vagina, and she told the obstetrician about it. The doctor said it was probably a yeast infection, and he gave her an over-the-counter vaginal cream to use for three days. The treatment cleared up her symptoms. I asked Shook whether she had developed more symptoms after the delivery, and she said that she hadn't noticed anything out of the ordinary.

In my office, the workup for a child with an autism spectrum disorder always includes a careful evaluation for CRC, as well as a diagnostic protocol for the possibility of Lyme disease. Let me explain why.

Back in the summer of 2003 when I was practicing in Wilton, Connecticut, the local health department reported that 54 percent of the town's families (total population about 18,000) had Lyme disease. That is a raging epidemic! Lyme disease is a bacterial infection spread through the bite of the blacklegged tick. It can affect different body systems, such as the nervous system, and the joints, skin, and heart. Although this youngster did not have any history of a tick bite or a rash, I checked anyway because I was "on a roll" having had six children with the diagnosis of autism consecutively test positive for Lyme disease. After the fourth confirmation, I had begun testing all children on the spectrum, and before I left Connecticut later that year I had nine consecutive autistic children test positive for Lyme disease. Unfortunately, I did not get to treat them all. Several of them went back to their pediatricians, who pooh-poohed the diagnosis because it did not meet the Centers for Disease Control (CDC) and Prevention's standard diagnostic criteria. But our laboratory testing, which is more sensitive and more specific than that recommended by the CDC, indicated the children had Lyme disease. Further testing also revealed that this youngster had Candida.

I treated the child for both CRC and Lyme disease. The first step I believe is to suppress the Candida *before* starting antibiotics, using antifungals drugs and probiotics, and nutrients for immune support with transfer factor extract and beta-glucans. And, since I also believe that the best-documented therapy for Lyme disease is combined antibiotics, I follow it with three different antibiotics, started one at a time and ultimately continued simultaneously, which can be different according to the patient's illness.

With testing we also determined that that Shook had Candida. Since I believe CRC should be treated as a sexually transmitted disease, we had to treat her husband too. As a very welcome postscript, this young child came back to life and by the time he was ready for first grade he was mainstreamed into a regular class, despite a pediatric neurologist telling the parents when the symptoms first developed that he would never be able to graduate from high school.

CLINICAL PEARL: Candida, Chemicals, and the Brain

Our federal agencies have failed to take a stand against a litany of toxic horrors at the expense of the health and safety of our children and their children, who will be even more impacted by an environment that is failing us. Getting pregnant without being really healthy is a major source of the decline in the health of our children and it's caused in large part by the decline in the quality of our food supply. And we cannot leave out keeping cigarettes on the market, mercury in dental fillings, fluoride in our water supplies, and fuel emissions far above achievable levels that underlie many illnesses and deaths.

There are bizarre changes occurring in male and female genitals, sexuality, and fertility. Girls are starting to menstruate at younger and younger ages; women are experiencing more infertility, premature births, and congenital malformations in their children. Boys are maturing later, with smaller-sized penises; men are experiencing dramatic decreases in the volume of semen, and in the number and quality of sperm cells. The term "endocrine disruptors" was coined by Theo Colburn, Ph.D., world-renowned scientist and founder of the Endocrine Disruption Exchange, and was rather quickly discovered to be related to many of the "new" chemicals that were poured out by the chemical industry under the great advertising slogan: "Better Living through Chemistry." Chemical exposures from industrial pollution, pesticides, and consumer products such as plastics, which are used in everything from baby bottles, nipples, and pacifiers to bottles and bags, can interfere with hormones that regulate the body's vital endocrine systems.

We doctors are still slowly poisoning our patients with our treatment solutions! Those changes were described by a Texas rancher as being so severe that if he had found similar changes in his herd of cattle, he would have slaughtered them and buried the bodies, and started a new herd from better genetic stock. I believe we now understand that most of these changes are not the result of damage to the genes, but rather to the change in the expression of the genetic material by the changes in the external environment.

What does this have to do with CRC? Our immune system is one of the targets for the damage brought about by all these toxic substances, and it functions as a second brain, without our thinking about it. It is critical to the prevention and eradication of any and all infections. Candida is one of the previously minor infections that have become a severe problem to many unsuspecting patients. As with many other infections, CRC can affect the brain's functions adversely, and does so frequently.

In my opinion, every parent, grandparent, babysitter, grade school teacher, and *every* physician should read the following, fascinating, and infuriating books:

- *Our Toxic World: Who Is Looking After Our Kids?* by Harold Buttram, M.D., and Richard Piccola. New Hope, PA: Foresight America for Preconception Care, 1996.
- *Our Stolen Future: Are We Threatening Our Fertility, Intelligence, and Survival?* by Theo Colburn. New York: Dutton, 1996.
- *Our Toxic World* by Doris Rapp, M.D. Buffalo, NY: Environmental Research Foundation, 2003.
- *Poisoned for Profit: How Toxins Are Making Our Children Chronically Ill* by Philip and Alice Shabecoff. White River Junction, VT: Chelsea Green Publishing, 2010.

BEHAVIORAL AND PSYCHIATRIC DISORDERS

CRC is one of many chronic infections that can have a major impact on psychiatric disorders that are otherwise unexplainable, including behavior problems in children. It can cause a vast array of nervous system symptoms such as irritability, extreme mood swings, hyperactivity, and problems with attention and concentration. In Peter's case, however, the origin of his Candida was Lyme disease.

Peter's Story

Peter, age eleven, a Connecticut resident, had been treated for Lyme disease with long-term antibiotics. In the mid-Atlantic area and in many other endemic areas for Lyme disease throughout the United States, the combination of Lyme disease and CRC is almost inevitable because treatment of Lyme disease is long-term antibiotics. Unfortunately, the guidelines for such treatment from the government and the Infectious Disease Society of America (IDSA) do not specify any preventive treatment to avoid the development of CRC.

As the first intervention for Peter, I prescribed a high dose of Diflucan with Phase 1 of my Anti-Yeast Diet. Research from Germany has shown that Diflucan, in addition to its antifungal activity, also suppresses the growth of Lyme disease organisms. By starting out with this antifungal drug, I significantly reduce the likelihood of Candida overgrowth from the long-term antibiotic regimen currently recommended by the International Lyme & Associated Disease Society (ILADS) for Lyme disease. Following a month of Diflucan, the antifungal was changed to nystatin, and a month later I switched to a bactericidal antibiotic. I often use this complex antibiotic protocol for treating both Lyme disease and CRC. I also placed Peter on high-dose probiotic therapy to keep healthy levels of good bacteria in his intestines.

Nutritionally, Peter needed support, much more than the rest of the population. I also suggested a high-quality multivitamin/mineral supplement supported by additional levels of antioxidants, including vitamins A, C, E, as well as selenium (ACES, as I call this group of supplements), as well as vitamin D and various minerals preferably as determined from testing of mineral levels in the red blood cells. In addition, I used various nutrients to supplement immune function including glutathione, lipoic acid, transfer factors, thymic proteins, essential fatty acids, and MPS (short for mucilaginous polysaccharides).

CLINICAL PEARL: Antibiotic Arsenal for Lyme Disease and Candida

At the current time, I use an arsenal of antibiotics from at least three different classes: bacteriostatic antibiotics, cyst-buster antibiotics, and bactericidal antibiotics. Started one by one in that order, with at least two-week intervals, each new prescription is added to the previous antibiotic and is continued until indicated by follow-up testing. While I find this triad approach most always proves successful, treating both Candida and Lyme disease simultaneously can be tricky and occasionally confounding.

I recently read about a case in which another Lyme-literate doctor was treating a patient, who had developed a severe Candida infection as a complication of the long-term but ineffective combined antibiotic therapy she was receiving for her Lyme disease. She had become resistant to treatment with Diflucan. (As I mentioned in Peter's case history, Diflucan often effectively suppresses the growth of both Candida and Lyme disease organisms, and as such is a valuable therapeutic tool.) In an attempt to treat his patient's Candida, the physician prescribed Vfend, the latest of the conazole-based drugs, and to the patient's and his surprise, her Lyme disease and Candida symptoms greatly improved.

BIPOLAR DISORDER

I have had three patients with severe bipolar disorder, all of whom had failed to achieve mental health and well-being following the pharmaceutical approach of mainstream psychiatry in America. Let me tell you briefly about them. Two of them were youngsters. As with other patients in this book, I am not using their real names, although my references to other scientists and physicians are all as accurate as I can make them.

Harry's Story

Harry was seven years old at his first visit. He was totally uncommunicative. He did not speak legibly, and there was no evidence that he heard anything that anyone said to him. He was difficult to control, and his mother was on the verge of her own breakdown. He was attending a special education school, and he had an aide assigned to him alone.

Sylvia, his mother, told me that he had been seen by twenty-one physicians (yes, that's right) in hospital emergency rooms and inpatient hospitals, and was currently on four (yes, four!) psychotropic drugs. According to the *Physicians' Desk Reference* (*PDR*), a standard source of drug information for physicians, only one of these drugs had been approved for use in children and two had "unknown" modes of action. When Harry was in the hospitals he was always in restraints, strapped down to the bed, and immobilized for his own protection.

I was still living and practicing in Connecticut at the time, and had just attended a post-graduate seminar at a local hospital on Lyme disease. I had learned that Lyme disease could cause mental illness, so I tested him for Lyme disease, and it was positive! He also had a history of chronic respiratory infections, with frequent antibiotic therapy, and had not taken probiotics or antifungals with the antibiotics.

I tested Harry for Candida and he was off the chart! I started him on treatment for both the Candida and Lyme infections, and he worsened, so his mother took him to one of the hospitals that he had been to previously. He had been on the medications and supplements for about a week. As usual, they sedated him and strapped him down. When he awoke, the doctors were going to sedate him again, but Sylvia said: "He looks different, please don't give him more medication." The doctors insisted, so this brave mother, trusting her maternal instincts, signed him out of the hospital against the doctors' advice.

As he recovered from his drug-induced stupor, she saw him for the first time in years as "being here." The aggravation of his symptoms had been a die-off reaction to both anti-infective agents. As mentioned earlier, this is a common occurrence when treating CRC and should be viewed as a good sign, despite the suffering.

The short of the story is that now, at least eight years later, Harry is attending a regular school, where he is doing well both socially and in his studies. I knew we were on the right track when he came into the office quietly, looking intently at his hand, which was held in a fist. His mother said, "Show Dr. Levin what you have." He opened his fist, looked me in the eye and said: "It's a bug, Dr. Levin." Sylvia and I cried and hugged each other, and then hugged Harry.

Milton's Story

My second bipolar patient was the father of Harry, the youngster I just told you about. Aha! you say, it was genetic. Well, you would be wrong. Harry was adopted. Milton, his adoptive father had been a successful lawyer, who had had a nervous breakdown and was on multiple medications. He had lost his job but was functional enough to eke out a living. With treatment for his CRC, I was able to get him off his drugs, but he was unable to pull himself together to stay on the restrictive diet and the large number of supplements required to maintain his remission, even though while on the program he felt "better than he had in years." So he never truly got well.

Molly's Story

My third psychotic patient was a teenager. She had been on multiple medications for two years, and in and out of mental hospitals multiple times. Her mother said that she had been given, "Every antipsychotic drug they had, except one." I never did find out which one, or why.

We talked about Molly's diet on the first visit, and as we all know, teenagers are picky eaters, who flaunt their newfound independence by eating a junk food diet. Well, between her diet and the typical terrible food in hospitals, she was overfed and undernourished.

During her last hospitalization, Molly and Molly's mother, Patricia, consulted with a group of specialists. The doctors told Molly and her mother that they were unable to find a suitable medication, so they were recommending electroconvulsive therapy (ECT), formerly known as electroshock. Molly's mother was horrified and signed her daughter out of the hospital.

Somehow Patricia learned about me, and brought Molly to see me. She had many abnormalities in her nutritional evaluation, and also had a raging Candida infection. I explained that her brain could not heal without the necessary nutrients. I gave her nutrient IVs and a strict diet, with many vitamins and minerals, and lots of fish oil along with heavy antifungal medications.

The three of us—Molly, Patricia, and me—were featured in a four-part documentary by health-advocate Gary Null, Ph.D., called *Healing Depression and Anxiety Naturally* (www.garynull.com). As Patricia says in that interview, "When I walked into the kitchen and heard her singing, I knew I had my daughter back."

CLINICAL PEARL: Omega-3 Fatty Acids and the Brain

Did you know that the dry weight of the human brain is approximately 70 percent fat? And that about two-thirds of that fat is identical to the biologically active omega-3 fatty acids found in fish oil? One of the great tragedies in industrialized countries today is that most kids do not get enough fish oil from their diets to foster optimum brain growth and development! In previous generations, cod liver oil was a standard supplement given to children as well as a source of argument between moms and kids. How did these mothers know? Why didn't modern doctors believe them? Infant feeding formulas have only recently begun to use omega-3 oils in their products!

In addition to supporting proper brain development, omega-3 fish oils are thought to fight depression and other mood disorders. They help the brain make neurotransmitters (brain chemicals) that facilitate communication between cells, including receptors for serotonin, a brain chemical that influences mood! Did you know that a study on depressed patients comparing selective serotonin reuptake inhibitors (SSRIs, widely prescribed antidepressants) against a placebo and fish oil supplement (2 grams per day) showed that the drugs gave some relief early, but that this effect did not last? Patients taking the placebo experienced little relief, but those taking the fish oil supplement were much better at the end of one year than either of the other groups (Nemets, *Am J Psychiatry,* 2002).

The building blocks for body repair must come from our outer environment. Because our bodies cannot produce omega-3 fatty acids, we must get these important substances from our diet. Omega-3 fatty acids are found predominately in cold-water fatty fish such as salmon, sardines, mackerel, herring, and albacore tuna, and in krill, squid, octopus, and marine algae. They are also available as supplements from these food sources.

Our children are being diagnosed with adult psychosis nomenclature—and for the most part it is just plain arbitrary. Daniel Amen, M.D., a child and adult psychiatrist who specializes in brain imaging, primarily by single-photon emission computerized tomography (SPECT) scan, accuses his fellow specialists of practicing "the only medical specialty that treats an organ without examining it."

On the wall in my office I have a quote by physicist Emerson Pugh that reads: "If the human brain were simple enough that we could understand it, we would be so simple [minded] that we couldn't understand it." That is the kernel of the wonderful idea behind the term "orthomolecular psychiatry," created by the two-time Nobel Prize winner and molecular biologist Linus Pauling, Ph.D. *Ortho* is from the Greek, meaning "right," or "straight," or "correct." You go to an *ortho*dontist to get your teeth straight, to an *ortho*pedist to get your feet straight, and to an *ortho*molecular physician to get the right molecules needed for your body to rebuild and repair itself. It is delusional thinking to expect that a foreign chemical—the product of human invention produced by a chemical manufacturer—can "fix" a brain that is not functioning properly! Omega-3 fatty acids are one of these essential building blocks for both the body and mind.

CHRONIC FATIGUE AND DEPRESSION

Paul, age eighteen, was tired all the time. He "ate right," did his best to exercise three times a week, and took vitamins, yet he had trouble getting out of bed in the morning. The first sign of a yeast infection in women is frequently vaginitis, then fatigue. Men, on the other hand, have fewer risk factors than women for CRC, as well as some different symptoms. Men don't take birth control pills! They don't get PMS, menstrual cramps, menstrual irregularities, polycystic ovaries, or endometriosis. This means that men must be even more conscious of the presence of the other triggers for developing CRC. Paul felt that something unexplained was zapping his energy, but what?

Paul's Story

I questioned Paul about the usual causes of excessive fatigue and depression in a healthy young man. He certainly appeared to be healthy. There was no significant family history that might explain his fatigue. He had no recent acute illnesses that might be going away gradually, no recent bleeding, no loss of sleep, no known exposure to anyone with a virus or other infection, no known exposure to mold or toxins at home or work, and no known allergies to foods or environmental triggers.

Paul was a senior in high school, and was often unable to attend because he would often faint without provocation. He had gone through the usual tilt-table testing by a neurologist who pronounced he had orthostatic hypotension, a form of low blood pressure that happens when you stand up from sitting or lying down. He gave Paul symptomatic medication that did not provide relief. After seeing an internist, another neurologist, and a psychiatrist, who offered him antidepressants as though he were neurotic, and then major antipsychotic medications, Paul was brought into my office in a wheelchair. I met him in the reception area and asked his caregiver to bring him into my office. Just starting up the wheelchair was enough to cause Paul to lose consciousness. And this is only half his case study!

Well, of course he was depressed! Who would not be? If he were psychotic, he might have come up with some sort of explanation about the police or little green men being after him. I told him that I would guarantee in writing that he did not have a deficiency of Prozac or Risperdol, two widely used antidepressants.

His past history was positive for a ruptured appendix when he was in his late teens, and had almost died. During the appendectomy, the surgeon had found a large abscess around the appendix, which required that Paul be hospitalized for ten days. He was given a massive amount of antibiotics—initially intravenously, and after a few days, orally—multiple times a day. Afterward, Paul developed diarrhea that was treated symptomatically, and gradually subsided. However, he confided, that since that time he had had irregular bowel habits with a lot of gurgling, gas, and a great deal more flatulence than pre-operatively.

During his physical exam, I found Paul's wound to be well healed, with no residual tenderness. His examination was otherwise unremarkable, except that he had severe dandruff. The problem had started a few weeks after his hospitalization and was reasonably well controlled with over-the-counter antidandruff shampoos. But because Paul didn't like the smell of the shampoos, he didn't use them regularly. He also had developed generalized dry skin with severe itching. He had seen a dermatologist, who diagnosed the condition as eczema and prescribed a cortisone-type cream that controlled those symptoms. (My dermatology professor told us that eczema is pronounced *X-zema* and the X stands for "unknown cause.")

Paul's stool was loaded with yeast and the Organic Acid Test confirmed a major colonization. I did give him symptomatic therapy as well (that is one of the important functions of a physician), yet it was not with drugs but with nutritional supplements. The supplements included a broad-based multiple vitamin/mineral supplement with extra vitamins A and D, a special fat-soluble form of vitamin B_1 (allithiamine), and magnesium taurate. I also gave him a high-potency probiotic supplement and the antifungal Diflucan. I put Paul on my Yeast-Free Diet and recommended large doses of probiotics and prebiotics to repopulate his gastrointestinal tract with healthy bacteria and increase his immune response.

Believe it or not, Paul's symptoms cleared and he was able to graduate with his class, and was accepted to college, where he enjoyed participation in athletics without fatigue and depression.

CLINICAL PEARL:
How to Avoid Candida as a Result of Surgery

Late in the 1980s, when I was still in my family practice but had already had my epiphany about integrative medicine and the inability to "fix" a patient by conventional medical means alone, I realized how poorly many of my patients were eating. It was long before the expression "junk food" became common usage. No doctors knew about the dangers of processed foods and harmful trans fats.

It was at a small study group, which got together four to six times a year (a planned cross-pollination of sorts, with many of the best minds in the nascent alternative medicine movement), that I introduced my concept of pre-operative care, or "pre-op" care. It was unanimously greeted with enthusiasm.

I recommended that for all elective (non-emergency) surgery every patient should have pre-op care to support the healing process and lessen any surgical discomfort and pain. I envisioned the pre-op would include a complete physical exam, laboratory testing, and nutritional evaluation, at least six weeks in advance of the surgery, so that a remedial program could be started to correct any abnormalities detected from the test results. Every patient would be counseled on the importance of eating a well-balanced and healthful diet, exercising, and taking extra zinc and vitamin C (nutrients that are essential for wound healing). Other recommendations would be tailored to the patient's test results. I envisioned this assessment would also identify minor addictions to such substances as sugar, caffeine, tobacco, and "party drugs." The withdrawal response is a major stress on the body, and is not the way to go into surgery, unless it is an emergency. This program was instituted at my facility in New York City and was written up in *Medical World News*, a now-defunct weekly publication that went to most practitioners in this country.

Today, "post-op" care is standard procedure in all hospitals. The nutritional value of hospital food remains inadequate in many facilities, as is the use of nutritional supplements. The peer-reviewed literature is full of reputable studies from many of the best medical centers about improved healing from such interventions. It is plain common sense, but common sense is a most uncommon thing in the world of medicine.

When antibiotics are administered to surgery patients, an antifungal like nystatin, as well as prebiotics and probiotics, must be prescribed along with a yeast-free diet. Ask your doctor or surgeon about incorporating these into your recovery plan.

FOOD ALLERGY ADDICTION AND OVERWEIGHT

Very often patients who present with CRC have food allergies and addictions. I find that the majority of these patients are almost always allergic and/or addicted to sugar and refined carbohydrates.

The McClarity's Story

Sugar is the root cause of many people's weight problems. Mr. and Mrs. McClarity and their two children were addicted to sweets and highly refined carbohydrate foods. The McClaritys are not alone. On average Americans consume 142 pounds of sugar per person each year, 68 percent of whom are either overweight or obese.

Food allergy is a common cause of cravings and overeating, although this connection is not always evident. It takes three days for a food to pass out of the body. You may not crave the allergic food the day you eat it, but as the food digests and begins to leave your body, you want more of it, and so the craving begins. By the third day, if you have not had the offending food, your body can react with almost any nasty symptom: fatigue, headache, anger, brain fog, joint pain, weight gain. In the same way as someone who is addicted to alcohol or drugs experiences a temporary high and suffers withdrawal symptoms when the substance is withdrawn, a person with an allergy to sugar or any other food (I have seen it happen with lettuce) will often experience similar reactions, causing him or her to "need" another fix. A delayed food allergy develops gradually over a period of months and even years. This is why delayed food allergies as opposed to rapid-onset severe food reactions are much more common and more difficult to recognize.

Although the McClarity family scenario is rarely seen in practice, I believe it is much more common than recognized. It is not unusual for family members to play "ping pong" with Candida. Yet despite the common denominator of CRC, it is my experience that each member has some unique manifestation of the infection, from athlete's foot to cradle cap and diaper rash, to psoriasis or brain fog. The reaction indicating CRC is appropriate to each age group.

CRC makes all allergic problems worse, especially when the addictive food is sugar, because the Candida organism requires sugar for its existence and growth. Somehow it communicates this to the appetite center of the host, which significantly increases the sugar-craving signals, setting up a continuing cycle.

I recommended the McClarity family begin Phase 1 of my Yeast-Free Diet. The first week was difficult as they withdrew from their sugar addiction. But they persisted and transitioned to Phase 2. By the time they reached Phase 3, they were all on their way to normal weight and enjoying their new bodies.

HYPERACTIVITY

Hyperactivity, inattention, impulsiveness, and other behavior problems in children are common manifestations of CRC. Children's small bodies can be particularly susceptible to the toxic byproducts produced by the Candida organism.

Rosie's Story

Rosie was about ten when she came to see me with her parents. I noticed that she could not sit still in her chair. Her mother confided that at night she would wake up and color the wallpaper with her crayons. She was very clever and played jokes on the family. One morning her father went into the bathroom, sat down, and slid to the floor. Rosie had oiled the toilet seat. Those things were mildly amusing, but her behavior in school was not. She was disruptive in class, pulled other girls' ponytails, threw spitballs at the boys, and often just walked around the classroom when the teacher was speaking.

Her parents had taken her for psychological testing and there wasn't anything seriously wrong, but the doctor suggested she go on Ritalin. This was very upsetting to her mother and she began looking for alternatives. A friend told her about me. I told her that I could promise Rosie "did not have a deficiency of Ritalin," but I knew that was how the previous doctor was going to treat her.

Rosie was a perfect example of a hyperactive child. She also had attention deficit hyperactivity disorder (ADHD). When I questioned her parents about her diet, they said, "Rosie craves sweet foods, and if we don't give them to her, she has a tantrum, and her behavior becomes more dramatic."

I asked whether she had been born with thrush in her mouth, and they said, "So that is what it is called. Yes, she did." And so, I suspected that her mother had CRC and passed it on to Rosie. I tested both of them using my Candida battery of tests.

I was concerned about the five days after taking Rosie off of sugary foods, and I suggested that her mother go on the diet first for a couple of weeks so they would not both be detoxing from sugar and wheat together.

I began by giving Rosie an antifungal and probiotic powder made for children. A month went by and her mother called. She said Rosie was feeling much better, but she needed some hand-holding as she weaned Rosie from sweet foods. Together, we were able to bring her through, and three months later she was a new child. Her teachers called Rosie's parents to school asking what had happened to exact the change. Rosie had become friendly, cooperative, and seemed to love reading and learning. What a great result!

CLINICAL PEARL:
Whatever Became of "Just Say 'NO!' to Drugs"?

Today's schoolchildren are suffering from man-made epidemics in comparison to 50 or 100 years ago. School nurses have shelves full of prescription drugs for conditions that were rare until recently. They administer anti-asthmatic drugs to kids in grammar school and treat ADHD with Adderall, an addictive stimulant composed of mixed amphetamine salts (speed-type drugs), which for some "unknown" reason seems to quiet down these kids. Another widely prescribed stimulant for ADHD, Ritalin, has the exact same mechanism of action as cocaine. It is slower to act, yet lasts longer. Hard to believe? Read it for yourself in the *Journal of the American Medical Association* (Vastag, JAMA 2001).

I find it particularly abhorrent when the latest and easiest way of treating children as patients is to drug them into submission. Especially considering that the proven short-term side effects of Adderall and Ritalin include nervousness, headaches, sleeplessness, depression, and decreased appetite, and their long-term side effects are unknown. This is an example of psychopharmacology at its worst. "What else is there to do?" you might ask, to which I would answer, "Find the cause of your child's symptom and correct it, instead of masking the problem with toxic drugs." Big Pharma now teaches the majority of classes for physicians after they graduate medical school than any other source! And it is for profit.

Whatever became of "Just Say No! to Drugs"? In the book *No More Ritalin* (1995), colleague Mary Ann Block, D.O., claims that the acronym ADHD really stands for "Another Doctor Handing Out Drugs"! If you want to learn a lot more about this travesty, go to https://secure.cchr.org/store/documentaries-and-dvds/industry-of-death.html, and feast on the facts.

INFERTILITY

Candida is a yeast condition that can impact fertility, as Nina and Philip Goldberg found out.

The Goldberg's Story

The Goldbergs had a fertility problem. Nina, age twenty-nine, had been checked by her gynecologist and was told there was no reason why she and her husband, Philip, should not be able to conceive. Nina had undergone the usual diagnostic testing, including a metabolic profile, speculum exam, Pap smear, pelvic sonogram (ultrasound), and a very uncomfortable probing of her fallopian tubes.

Nina mentioned that she had been taking birth control pills for at least fifteen years, starting in high school. At that time they had been prescribed for severe pain associated with her menstruation. She continued taking the birth control pills for pain when she went off to college. I asked her whether she had ever taken antibiotics during all those years on the pill.

Nina readily recalled several instances. In her sophomore year, she had been diagnosed with sinusitis and was treated with several weeks of tetracycline. She remembered developing gastrointestinal symptoms as a result. Her mother had given her some Kaopectate, an antacid and anti-diarrhea medication, and she recovered. A short time later, however, she returned to the gynecologist as she had developed a vaginal discharge that was caused by the antibiotics. Nina's doctor gave her an over-the-counter vaginal yeast treatment that she took for three days, which cleared up the problem.

On further questioning, Nina recalled that she had also had a sinus problem during her junior year in high school that had finally cleared with antibiotics. More recently, her gastrointestinal symptoms had returned, and she was told that she had gluten sensitivity. (Gluten is a protein found in many grains including wheat, rye, barley, and oats that can cause bloating, abdominal discomfort, and pain.) She went on a gluten-free diet and felt much better.

CLINICAL PEARL: Gluten and Thyroid Antibodies

There is a common belief among non-endocrinologists that Hashimoto's disease, an autoimmune disorder that affects the thyroid, is of unknown cause. Yet, nearly 50 percent of those who are diagnosed with the condition by the presence of autoantibodies (antibodies that in these cases are directed against the thyroid gland) also have gluten antibodies. This finding suggests some type of molecular mimicry is involved; the antibodies against gluten attack something in the thyroid that is molecularly so similar to gluten that those antibodies bind to it by mistake, and inflammation results.

Based on this last bit of information regarding her gluten sensitivity, I tested Nina's thyroid function. I measured the speed of her reflexes on a Thyroflex machine (invented by dear friend Konrad Kail, N.D.). Her reflexes were slow, a characteristic finding in patients with hypothyroidism (underactive thyroid). I then sent a blood sample to the lab for thyroid testing. Her blood tested on the low side of normal for free T3 and free T4, two hormones that control how quickly the body burns calories and uses energy.

I asked Nina to test herself for an underactive thyroid by keeping track of her body temperature for five days. This entailed taking her body temperature three times a day, keeping a temperature log, and including her morning pulse rate before getting out of bed. An average temperature of 98.6°F or lower indicates low thyroid function. Nina's average body temperature was below 97.7°F. (For more information on this treatment for an underactive thyroid, go to www.wilsonssyndrome.com.)

Based on several other events in her medical history, I ordered a complete Organic Acid Test (OAT) from Great Plains Laboratory. It confirmed the presence of a significant systemic Candida problem, plus abnormally low levels of vitamins B_6 and B_{12} as well as several markers for impaired function of the Krebs cycle, a group of reactions that helps supply the body with energy. (Vitamins B_3, B_6 and B_{12}, magnesium, manganese, and thyroid hormone are the main catalysts in the Krebs cycle.)

I then asked Nina to take an Adrenal Stress Index (ASI) test to evaluate her adrenal gland function. The adrenal gland is a small gland on the tip of the kidney. The medulla, or inner part of the gland, regulates the immediate stress reactions in the body by producing epinephrine, the so-called "fight, fright, and flight hormone," while the outer cortex of the gland assists the testes and ovaries by producing dozens of hormones based upon the cholesterol molecule. (Remember the days when all cholesterol was "bad"?) Pregnenolone and dehydroepiandrosterone (DHEA) are steroid hormones and precursors to the sex hormones: estrogen and progesterone in women, and testosterone in men. By a slightly different pathway, all the adrenal corticosteroids are also produced, including cortisone, hydrocortisone, and aldosterone. Without sound endocrine function, you can pretty much count on your fertility becoming affected in some way.

The ASI test involves taking four saliva specimens throughout a single day. Nina's hydrocortisone and pregnenolone levels were low, indicating a "stressed out" pattern, and the test also identified elevated gluten antibodies in her saliva. Gluten sensitivity often causes adrenal stress and fatigue, and can also participate in autoimmune thyroiditis (Hashimoto's thyroiditis). I use Diagnos-Techs for this test.

The next visit Nina came with her thirty-two-year-old husband, Philip. I reviewed these findings, and although I could not promise that she would get pregnant, I felt that we had identified the majority of her metabolic abnormalities, all of which were correctable to some degree. None of these conditions had been tested by her gynecologist.

Because Nina's Candida infection had begun many years ago in high school, I was particularly aggressive in my treatment protocol. I started her on my Yeast-Free Diet, paying special attention to avoid prepared and packaged foods, using only fresh and organic foods, prepared at home. To support her body's fighting armamentarium, I gave her intravenous nutrients that included a broad spectrum of vitamin and minerals with the ACES antioxidants (vitamins A, C, E, and the trace mineral selenium), and a mixture of amino acids. I also prescribed a high-potency probiotic and a one-month supply of Diflucan in higher doses than many other doctors might do. I also urged Nina to start an exercise program.

I started Philip on a similar protocol for men. Like most of my patients, Philip had a basic blood profile that was unremarkable, and he charted his temperatures, which were normal as well. (This is why most patients are misdiagnosed. The "usual and customary" tests are usually okay!) I also ordered a semen analysis at Philip's first visit; the sperm count was fine, and their motility and morphology were also adequate. It took over three weeks to get the result of the yeast culture, and it was negative. There were no bacteria or white blood cells to indicate an infection. I then knew that Nina's health would be most important.

Since Nina's body temperature chart was well below the optimum 98.6°F (the temperature at which most of the body's metabolic functions work at their best), I started her on a synthetic time-released form of T3, twice a day, at exactly twelve hours apart, and incrementally increased the dose every day. By the second menstrual flow after starting the protocol, Nina reported that for the first time in her life she had not experienced some kind of discomfort with her monthly period!

And, believe it or not, the Goldbergs then went on their spiritual journey together, and they were rewarded with a hard-won pregnancy, without all the gadgetry and surgery. Nina delivered at home, in her bathtub, with a midwife. Of course, I wish that I could always see such results, but every such success is a special gift for me, as well as my patients.

CLINICAL PEARL: Infertile "Couples"

I want to interject an important objection to many doctors' evaluation of "infertile women." That diagnosis is not justified unless the father's health has been considered and carefully evaluated by testing. Until then, the proper diagnosis should be "infertile couple." The first person from the couple that goes to the doctor is usually the female, and many doctors go through an extensive (and expensive), incredibly uncomfortable, and occasionally risky evaluation of the woman, before looking at the possibility of the male's contribution.

It is much easier and less expensive to "rule out" the man as the cause of the failure to conceive. All that is involved for him is the examination of a specimen of seminal fluid from an ejaculation. (For those whose religious law may prohibit such a collection method, there are alternatives.) In some cases, the man may also require a digital rectal exam, which involves the physician's inserting a finger into the rectum to evaluate the prostate gland. It is still far less invasive and expensive, and less painful than the full exam for infertility that must be done for a complete evaluation of the woman's contribution to the problem.

Normal findings from microscopic, chemical, and bacterial analyses of the sperm are considered adequate, but hear this: in my opinion, an additional separate culture for Candida from the same specimen of sperm should be a further requirement! When Candida is present in large amounts, it may grow in a standard culture medium, but small amounts in an individual ejaculation may be missed if a special culture medium is not employed in the lab. This specific culture must be special ordered in many labs. Dividing a single specimen into two parts is easily done in the doctor's office.

IRRITABLE BOWEL SYNDROME

Libby, age forty-three, had disturbing irritable bowel symptoms: gas with burping and belching, gaseous distention of her abdomen that sometimes caused her to look pregnant, and gas from below that had a peculiar sweet foul smell which was extremely embarrassing to her. Libby was so self-conscious she rarely went out in public.

Libby's Story

Irritable bowel is the wastebasket term for a combination of symptoms that include those enumerated above, as well as irregularity in frequency and consistency of the bowel movements, which can vary from very loose to diarrhea, to relatively normal, to very hard and difficult to pass, to severe constipation. Frequently, these problems are associated with constant discomfort migrating around in the abdominal area, gurgling sounds, and occasional severe spasms of pain from the intestines. Gastrointestinal tract symptoms are a major component of the yeast problem. The presence of abdominal distention, particularly below the belt line, is a frequent indicator of the presence of yeast overgrowth, especially in females. No patient with symptoms like these should be treated without having a stool examination to determine which kinds of living entities are occupying the intestinal tract. The gut can also have a great deal of disturbance when normal healthy bacteria are not strong enough to keep out unhealthy organisms, and those organisms can produce any of the previous symptoms.

Irritable bowel syndrome (IBS) has many other causes besides infection. It turned out that Libby did indeed have an infection, but it wasn't just bacterial. She had a severe infection with Candida, which was confirmed when I sent her stool to the laboratory for a culture.

The lab not only grew bacteria but also a heavy load of yeast. I also asked the lab to do a special kind of parasite test since it had not found parasites in her stool sample. Intestinal parasites are a common cause of IBS, which can sometimes develop into inflammatory bowel disease, or IBD, a more serious and dangerous kind of illness.

Sure enough, as I expected, Libby's parasite test came back from the laboratory with a heavy growth of an intestinal parasite known as *Blastocystis hominis*. *B. hominis* is considered to be a relatively benign intestinal parasite. It does not cause severe symptoms like amoebic dysentery or giardiasis, but it does interfere with normal bowel function and can cause abdominal pain and other gastrointestinal complaints. I prescribed Nizoral for the blastocystosis, a great discovery I had read about long ago in a short letter to a major medical journal. Somehow or other, the doctor who wrote the letter had discovered that Nizoral was effective against infection with *B. hominis* as well as Candida. I have used it for many years since with great success. It helped Libby to change from a miserable IBS sufferer to a happy, healthy woman.

At that time I also recommended Libby take a number of carminative herbs to help dispel the gas, bloating, and indigestion. These included ajwain seed (*Trachyspermum ammi*) and basil (*Ocimum basilicum*), among others. I also prescribed an over-the-counter aluminum-free antacid to help temporarily neutralize the acid. This type of antacid does not lead to serious problems, as many acid-suppressing medications do. Libby then went on my Yeast-Free Diet. In one month, she was feeling much better. In three months, I retested her and her tests came back free of parasites and Candida.

CLINICAL PEARL:
Why You Should Not Take Acid-Suppressing Drugs

Millions of Americans suffering from heartburn, acid reflux, gastroesophageal reflux disease, or other acid-related problem take acid-suppressing medications known as proton pump inhibitors (PPIs). Prilosec, Prevacid, Protonix, Tagamet, and other PPIs work by blocking production of a powerful stomach acid called hydrochloric acid (HCl). Yet, HCl plays a number of critical roles in the breakdown and digestion of foods.

The digestion of chunks of food into smaller bits and pieces begins in the mouth with an enzyme in the saliva called salivary amylase. Its job is to break down starch (and other complex carbohydrates) into sugars, a major source of fuel for the body and brain. This breakdown of starch and carbohydrate continues in the stomach, where HCl and an enzyme known as pepsin combine to break down protein foods into smaller bits and pieces. These protein fragments eventually become amino acids, the building blocks of all proteins in the body. The stomach empties into the small intestine and even with food in it, these stomach secretions are very acid. The stomach is designed to hold undiluted HCl (just a little of which, if spilled on a rug, would burn it).

The rest of the intestinal tract, however, is not similarly protected. As a result, when the stomach empties its acid contents into the small intestine, the intestinal lining, or mucous membrane, gets irritated and weeps an alkaline solution to dilute and neutralize the acid. At the same time that the mucous membrane is triggered into activity, messenger molecules are secreted that tell the pancreas to release its digestive enzymes, which help digest protein, fat, as well as starch. The pancreatic juices are also very alkaline.

The same shock of acid also triggers the gallbladder to empty its contents of bile into the small intestine. Because fat particles tend to clump together, the body uses this bile along with lipase, an enzyme from the pancreas, to dissolve these large clumps into fatty acid droplets so that the body can absorb and utilize them. In infancy, fats are necessary for normal brain development, and throughout life they provide energy and support growth. All this is triggered by stomach acid. If HCl is lacking in the stomach, it doesn't produce this cascade of digestive response!

The entire digestive process requires this jolt of HCl. Without it your ability to properly digest food is impaired. If you fail to digest your food properly, you will be unable to absorb many of the valuable nutrients your body needs to function normally. Not only do you lose absorbing the nutritional value of the food, but you also risk absorbing particles of incompletely digested food that are too big yet manage to get through anyway. Because the body recognizes these particles as foreign, it causes an inflammatory reaction in the wall of the intestine. When the wall of the intestine becomes inflamed, it also becomes more porous, which allows more intestinal contents to be absorbed that otherwise should be evacuated.

In addition, when there is not enough HCl in the stomach, all kinds of harmful microorganisms (e.g, Candida, *Helicobacter pylori*, *Clostridium difficile*, etc.) that are swallowed all the time and should be killed in the stomach's resting acid, get through to the small and large intestines where they find a much more comfortable place to live. A healthy stomach would have kept them out.

PPIs are among the most commonly prescribed drugs in the United States. And while they can provide temporary digestive relief, they carry significant risks for good reason.

ITCHING

Sally, age thirty-three, and her husband, Richard, age thirty-five, are a perfect example of how CRC can be transferred between partners during oral sex (kissing mouth to mouth or mouth to genitals). It can be transmitted during genital sex and by sharing of towels, sheets, and generally careless contacts. Therefore, when the Candida organism is present in one partner, both partners should be treated simultaneously.

Sally and Richard's Story

While Sally and Richard each experienced itching in the genital or anal area, the itching may occur anywhere, with or without a rash, although constant scratching produces a rash. Sally was also taking birth control pills, which can cause an allergic reaction such as itching and increase the susceptibility of the vaginal lining to Candida.

There can be many different infectious causes of vaginitis and pruritus ani (the medical term for itching that occurs around the anus). But because the odds were great that this was CRC, as itching is the major complaint, I started the couple on oral and topical therapies. I prescribed nystatin for internal treatment of the yeast and recommended one of several over-the-counter topical antifungal creams, ointments, or sprays. Again, depending on the presence or absence of gastrointestinal symptoms, the specific prescription agents can be guessed prior to the final diagnosis, or if the physician has the proper microscope, the discharge or scraping of the affected areas can be evaluated at the time of the visit and a definitive diagnosis may be made. In either of the partners, a characteristic rash with a sharp red margin and small red dots outside of the margin can be diagnostic as well. It is appropriate for the clinician to *assume* that what one partner has is the same as the other for initial therapy! The results of testing on both patients should be reviewed at the follow-up visits, as well as the response to therapy.

MENSTRUAL DISORDERS AND LOW LIBIDO

Marilyn, a vital thirty-year-old recently married woman, came to see me because she had a fungus under her toenail, ten pounds she could not lose, chronic menstrual problems, and low libido (in that order). She thought she was finished with passion at age thirty.

Marilyn's Story

Marilyn had been living in Florida, a place where mold thrives because of the humidity, so I was not surprised by Marilyn's symptoms. She also said that she had been living a lascivious lifestyle, drinking wine, eating a high-carbohydrate diet, and before losing her libido, enjoying an active sex life with her new husband. She was worried.

Being a very attractive, well-dressed woman, it was obvious looking at her that appearance was important to her. Her major complaint when coming in was the toe fungus! She said that she didn't feel comfortable wearing open-toed shoes, had been to many doctors about the fungus, was given antibiotics and drugs that could have caused liver damage, and still had the fungus.

I asked Marilyn if there was anything else she would like me to treat. She said that she had gained ten pounds and could not take them off, even though she spent an hour in spin class four times a week. She asked if I could help her lose the pounds. And as I questioned her further, she said that she had irregular periods, and had completely lost her libido.

I did some blood and stool tests and found that Marilyn had CRC. We began treatment for the CRC with my Yeast-Free Diet. I asked Marilyn if she was willing to remove all carbohydrates from her diet, plus vinegar, alcoholic beverages, dried herbs, and tea and coffee. She said, "Yes."

Next came the supplement list: a probiotic, oil of oregano drops and capsules (the oil she applied directly to her nail three times daily), olive leaf extract, and grapefruit seed extract. She was willing to do this to clear the Candida that had spread to her toe.

I explained that she had had the fungus for a while, and it would not disappear overnight. It would probably take around three months. She wasn't happy about that, but agreed to stay with the program for that period. We made monthly appointments.

One month later, when Marilyn came back, she looked younger. Her skin was clear and bright and her hair seemed to shine in a way that it hadn't when we first met. She said that she had had her first normal menstrual cycle in years, and her "feminine feelings were returning." However, her fungus had not changed. Another month went by, and she kept her next appointment, even though she still had not lost any weight and her fungus hadn't budged. She seemed disheartened, and I reminded her that there was still one month to go. Although she wasn't hungry, she was bored with the limited foods she was permitted to eat. I asked her if she had cheated on the diet. She said, "No."

Two weeks later Marilyn called. "My nail fell off!" she exclaimed. "The fungus is gone." But, she still hadn't lost the weight. I asked her not to go off the diet, because if she did, the fungus might return. I promised that when I saw her next I would give her more foods to eat. When I saw Marilyn two weeks later, she was ten pounds thinner.

"How did it happen?" I asked.

"Almost overnight," she said. "On Wednesday, I suddenly had to urinate several times during the day. On Thursday morning, when I put my clothes on, I thought they felt loose. I urinated more than usual on Thursday, too. Then on Friday morning, I weighed myself, and I couldn't believe my eyes. The ten pounds were gone! I am never going off this diet!"

The yeast had caused Marilyn's body to retain ten pounds of extra fluids. She had to kill off the yeast before she could lose the weight.

URINARY TRACT INFECTIONS

For women like Cynthia, one of the first signs of CRC is a recurring urinary tract infection (UTI). You may remember that this twenty-seven-year-old woman came to see me with a long history of urinary tract infections that had often kept her out of school and at times even required hospitalization. Cynthia and her doctor were unable to get her UTIs under control despite a litany of medical tests and treatments that included an intravenous pyelogram (x-ray of the urinary tract), an MRI scan of the structure of her urinary tract, a cystoscopy exam (procedure used to examine the lining of the bladder and urethra), and multiple courses of antibiotics.

Cynthia's Story

When Cynthia came to see me, my first question was, "Have you ever had a vaginal yeast infection?" "Always," she replied, "That's part of my life. It's really terrible and it's so bad that I don't have a social life anymore, because I feel so miserable."

I did my routine evaluation, which confirmed that she did indeed have a chronic urinary tract infection. We identified the organism and had the bug tested for sensitivities to determine which antibiotics would be most effective against her particular bacterial infection of the kidneys and bladder. However, before I started Cynthia on yet another round of antibiotics, I said to her: "Has anyone ever talked to you about getting your yeast infection under control?" She replied that she had mentioned it to several doctors and they all gave her something to take as vaginal therapy—the old trio: douches, creams, and suppositories. They may have worked temporarily but the yeast came back, so she had given up.

I explained to Cynthia what I had learned from C. Orian Truss, M.D., about Candida and its connection to many common health disorders. I suggested that we try to clear her intestinal tract of the yeast before we try again to get rid of the urinary infection. "How do you know I have it in my intestines?" she asked. I said: "Well, I know but if you want to prove it, that's not a bad idea." So I ordered a stool test and sure enough it came back from the laboratory with a heavy growth of Candida and the intestinal parasite, *Blastocystis hominis*. I had learned about an effective treatment for blastocystosis with the medication Nizoral, one of the conazole-based drugs used for treating resistant yeast problems. I said: "I think you are going to really have a major improvement just from getting your intestines cleared up."

So Cynthia began the program with my Yeast-Free Diet, the anti-fungal Nizoral, a high-potency probiotic supplement, and several nutritional supplements to enhance her immune system, including thymus extract, transfer factor extract, and beta-glucan. Knowing that I had taken care of the systemic infection, I added topical treatments to give Cynthia local relief more quickly. I suggested she use douches, creams, ointments, suppositories, or sprays, depending on her preference and what her local druggist carried or recommended.

When I saw her a few weeks later she was very happy. Cynthia exclaimed, "It didn't come back this time. Is it going to come back?" I said, "Well, I certainly hope we got it under control, but now we have to deal with the urinary infection and that requires antibiotics."

By this time I had received the antibiotic sensitivity report, which indicated her bacterium was not the usual *Escherichia coli* (*E. coli*), a type of bacteria commonly found in the intestines that cause urinary infections, but a more resistant bacterium known as *Klebsiella*. Using the test results, I found that the usual medications for run-of-the-mill UTIs would not be effective. Her infection required a different kind of antibiotic, one of the newer, more targeted antibiotics. I gave her an aggressive course of antibiotic therapy and felt that we had a pretty good chance of getting the urinary infection under control.

Throughout Cynthia's treatment, she continued taking the probiotics. In addition to the nutritional supplements and immune enhancers prescribed earlier, I added a prebiotic supplement to help the probiotics grow and flourish. I discontinued the systemic antifungal and replaced it with nystatin, which is not absorbed from the gut and therefore does not challenge the liver.

Cynthia felt better and better. She came in really radiant on one of her visits and I said, "What's going on?" and she said, "Dr. Levin you got me in trouble." "How's that?" I asked. She said, "Well, you know I didn't have any social life and now I've been dating, and right now I'm dating two men and I can't make up my mind which one I like best!" I said, "That's really too bad, you'll just have to suffer through," and she laughed.

We continued with a reduced dosage of both the antibiotic and antifungal, and continued with protection for her bladder from her usual *E. coli* infections by giving her U-Tract, a nutrient (mannose) that coats the bladder so that the *E. coli* bacteria are unable to get a foothold and just pass through the entire urinary tract. I saw Cynthia again after New Year's and this time she had an engagement ring that she proudly showed me. I said, "Well, when did you get that? It's great news. Congratulations!" I then listened as she told me about her New Year's Eve with one of the two men that she had been dating—the one who she thought she really liked the best.

They started the evening at some parties where they drank wine and had various canapés, sweet pastries, and various appetizers on bread, and she thoroughly enjoyed them. Then they went for a lovely dinner and had more appetizers, candied yams with their main meal, wine and champagne, and desserts. They ended up at a midnight party once again drinking more champagne to toast the New Year, and then they went home and made passionate love. It was wonderful and they fell asleep together.

During the night Cynthia was awakened because she had wet the bed! That's right, she urinated in her sleep! She told me that she had been a bed-wetter as a child until the age of thirteen and that her family had tried all kinds of treatments. She related that her mother had been a "health nut" and had given her brewer's yeast at a very young age, and for a long time. Brewer's yeast is a healthful food derivative that is high in vitamins and many minerals (but, it is yeast after all). She had finally grown out of her bedwetting.

After not having wet the bed for all those years, what had happened was that she broke all the rules of the yeast-free, sugar-free, anti-Candida diet, all at once. She re-triggered a severe allergic reaction that resurrected her dormant target organ—her bladder. Lo and behold! Cynthia's whole bladder problem was tied to a chronic Candida infection, and the cross-reactive allergy to brewer's yeast.

One common manifestation of long-standing Candida infection in children (and in adults as well) is a severe allergy to other forms of yeast, such as brewer's yeast used to make beer, wine, and vinegar, and baker's yeast used to make bread, pastries, and other raised baked goods. It was unusual to produce bed-wetting in a grown woman, but I am sure there are many children with bed-wetting problems that are also related to food allergies, and very possibly to yeast overgrowth and yeast allergy as a result of the repeated antibiotic treatments for their urinary tract infections, recurrent ear infections, or sinusitis with or without bronchitis.

So Cynthia's problem had come full-circle and was finally solved!

CLINICAL PEARL: Attention All Females

All females are susceptible to urinary tract infections because of their anatomy—specifically, the close proximity of the urethra to the anus and the short distance from the urethral opening to the bladder.

When stool is passed that is contaminated with yeast, the organisms may stay on the outside of the anus in the cleft of tissue between the cheeks of the buttocks, especially if the area is not scrupulously cleaned. That area is warm, dark, and moist so the yeast can live there for a while (and that's true for both men and women). However, for a woman it is more important because the opening of the vagina is only about an inch and a half from the opening of the anus. It, too, is in an area that is warm and dark and moist, so proper feminine hygiene should be taught to children very early. Girls and women should always wipe from front to back—never from back to front.

LEVIN'S LAWS

As you have been reading in this book, Candida is a powerful infection that wreaks havoc on the immune system and many bodily functions. I hope that you understand how CRC may be affecting your health, and what is necessary to do to rid your body of the infection. Keep in mind what you've learned and always be proactive in the prevention of CRC by following Levin's Laws.

- Never take antibiotics without also taking antifungals and probiotic supplements. Make these healing nutrients part of your treatment regimen.
- Never let anyone tell you that a mild case of vaginitis is "normal," just because so many women have this condition. If a physician says that to you, give him or her a copy of this book and if it is refused or ignored, find another doctor.
- Never take birth control pills without also reducing the foods in your diet that encourage Candida to grow.
- Use cortisone-type drugs only in emergencies or in very small doses to support worn out adrenals.
- Avoid taking medications that suppress stomach acid.
- Drastically reduce your intake of refined and processed foods—especially sugar!

Conclusion

This book may be the most important health advice you have ever read. We know that it sounds very complicated, so we want to simplify it for you. If, after reading this book, you feel that any of the Candida-related maladies are affecting your life or the lives of loved ones—run, don't walk, to a physician who can help.

Dr. Levin now practices in the District of Columbia. If you can, please come to his office to be treated. If you cannot get to see Dr. Levin, contact the American Academy of Environmental Medicine (AAEM) and they will find a doctor in your area who can help you. (Contact information for Dr. Levin and the AAEM can be found in the Resource's section.)

This is your bottom line:

- You need to detoxify and rebuild your immune system.
- You need to go on the Yeast-Free Diet in this book.
- You need to take nutrients and probably some antifungal drugs to restore your body to normal health.

You can be well again. Now you have the awareness. Time to do the work. Both Dr. Levin and Dr. Gare wish you a pleasant journey back to optimal health. You can do it! It happens every day.

Resources

Food and Products

Celtic Sea Salt
4 Celtic Dr.
Arden, NC 28704
Phone: 800-867-7258
Website: www.celticseasalt.com

Goat Cream Cheese
Meyenberg Goat Milk Products
P.O. Box 934
Turlock, CA 95381
Phone: 800-891-GOAT (4628)
Website: www.meyenberg.com

Herbamare
A. Vogel
313 Iron Horse Way
Providence, RI 02908
Email: http://cs.bluemarblebrands.com/contactus/Pages/default.aspx
Website: www.herbamare.us

Tanalbit
Intensive Nutrition Inc.
1972 Republic Avenue
San Leandro, CA 94577
Phone: 800-333-7414
Website: www.intensivenutrition.com

U-Tract
Progressive Labs Inc.
1701 W. Walnut Hill Lane
Irving, TX 75038
Phone: 800-527-9512
Website: www.progressivelabs.com

Whey Protein Powder
Solgar
500 Willow Tree Road
Leonia, NJ 07605
Phone: 877-765-4272
Website: www.solgar.com

Xylitol
The Sweet Life
241–245 Oak Park Drive, Suite B
Douglaston, NY 11362
Phone: 516-759-2140
Website: www.perfectsweet.com

Finding a Doctor Who Treats Candida

Warren M. Levin, M.D.
National Integrated Health Associates
5225 Wisconsin Avenue, NW, Suite 402
Washington, DC 20015
Phone: 202-237-7000
Website: www.nihadc.com or www.warrenmlevinmd.org

Fran Gare, N.D.
Office of Integrative Medicine
635 Madison Avenue, 4th Floor
New York, NY 10022
Phone: 212-277-4406
Website: www.frangare.com

American Academy of Environmental Medicine
6505 E. Central Avenue, Suite 296
Wichita, KS 67206
Phone: 316-684-5500
Website: www.aaemonline.org

Laboratory Testing

Diagnos-Techs
19110 66th Ave S, Bldg G
Kent, Washington 98032
Phone: 800-878-3787
Website: www.diagnostech.com

Doctor's Data
3755 Illinois Avenue
St. Charles, IL 60174
Phone: 800-323-2784
Website:www.doctorsdata.com

Genova Diagnostics
63 Zillicoa Street
Asheville, NC 28801
Phone: 800-522-4762
Website: www.gdx.net

Great Plains Laboratory Inc.
11813 W. 77th Street
Lenexa, KS 66214
Phone: 800-288-0383
Website: www.greatplainslaboratory.com

Index

About the Authors

Warren M. Levin, M.D., opened the first alternative and integrative medical practice in New York City in 1974. Known as the East Coast Dean of Alternative Medicine, he was the first to scientifically document the link between Candida-related complex and parasites. Dr. Levin is listed in *Who's Who in American Medicine, Who's Who in America,* and *Who's Who in the World,* and was named in 2010 as a Top Doctor in America in Family and Integrative Medicine. He practices at National Integrative Health Associates in Washington, D.C.

Fran Gare, N.D., is a clinical nutritionist and naturopathic physician who has authored or co-authored six best-selling books, including *The Sweet Miracle of Xylitol* (2012), *Dr. Atkins' New Diet Cookbook* (2000), *The Mandells' It's Not Your Fault You're Fat* (1983), and *Dr. Atkins' Diet Revolution* (1981). Dr. Gare was Director of Nutrition at the Atkins Center for Complementary Nutrition, New York City, and Director of Natural Medicine at Miami Heart Hospital, where she also served as the on-camera Nutrition Expert correspondent for CBS in Miami. Dr. Gare appears frequently on national TV and radio and in print. You can read her articles in *Glow,* the online beauty magazine (www.glowbeautymag.com), where she is Nutrition Editor, or visit her at the Office of Integrative Medicine in New York.